# The GIFT of HEALING

## A Legacy of Hope

# The GIFT of HEALING

# HEALING

## A Legacy of Hope

# BEATRICE C. ENGSTRAND, M.D.

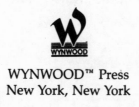

WYNWOOD™ Press
New York, New York

This book is autobiographical, and real names of institutions have been retained. Names of persons, however, have been changed in some instances to protect the privacy of individuals.

Library of Congress Cataloging-in-Publication Data
Engstrand, Beatrice C.
  The gift of healing : a legacy of hope / Beatrice C. Engstrand.
    p.    cm.
  ISBN 0-922066-31-0 : $16.95
    1. Engstrand, Beatrice C.—Health.  2. Palate—Tumors—Patients—United States—Biography.  3. Palate—Surgery—Patients—United States —Biography.  4. Surgery, Plastic—Patients—United States—Biography. 5. Neurologists—United States—Biography.  I. Title.
RD662.E54   1990
362.1′96994315′0092—dc20
[B]                                                                89-29844
                                                                      CIP

Copyright © 1990 by Beatrice C. Engstrand
Published by WYNWOOD™ Press
New York, New York
Printed in the United States of America

*To my mother,*
*whose love is a constant inspiration*

*To my father,*
*who supported both of us*

*To my brother,*
*Wende and Rachel, Aunt Augusta,*
*and Cousin Stokes with love*

*To my university and medical school*
*for having faith in me*

# The GIFT of HEALING

## A Legacy of Hope

# Chapter One

It was a crisp fall Friday, and I was bubbling over with excitement at the end of a tough week in my first year of medical school. Though I was physically exhausted, my spirits were soaring because I had just completed the next to last of a grueling series of written examinations, and had received honors on an earlier round of tests. I walked the few blocks from the Medical College of Pennsylvania (MCP) to my apartment in Philadelphia's Germantown section savoring my progress toward the dream of becoming a physician.

It had been a long time since, as a child growing up in Massapequa, New York, I had first heard the call to healing. It pushed me to excel in high school, and I had gone to Lehigh in the fall of 1978 for two years of the much-coveted six-year accelerated program with MCP. Now, though, at twenty, younger than most of my medical classmates who already had degrees, I found that Lehigh's courses and professors had prepared me well. I not only could keep up with my studies but had time to make friends and even to listen to classmates who suggested my nomination for class president. This success, however, was tempered by some very real worries.

One year earlier, in May 1979, at the end of my freshman year at Lehigh, an oral surgeon had operated on the roof of my mouth to excise what he told me was a small cyst. After the operation, in which part of my hard palate was removed, the surgeon reported that the lump had been mucoepidermoid cancer, but that he had removed the entire malignant growth. I returned to campus on schedule for the first summer session, despite constant headaches and a stuffy nose caused by the surgery. Even though I wore a prosthesis to cover the hole cut in the roof of my mouth, much of what I ate and drank spilled out through my nostrils, and I was annoyed and embarrassed.

The pain continued, and I decided to seek a second opinion from a head-and-neck surgeon, Dr. Robert Karik of Columbia-Presbyterian Medical Center. Though I remained home on Long Island for the second summer session, the next year at Lehigh went well. Then, a year after the initial surgery, the pain intensified and my vision dimmed. Dr. Karik, then affiliated also with Yale–New Haven Memorial Hospital, recommended a biopsy to determine if more cancer was present.

All this was far from my mind as I headed home on this bright October 3, 1980. Filled with the satisfaction of at last being a physician in training, I rushed up the stairs of my apartment building to tell the good news to my mother, Claudia, who had been staying with me since the biopsy. She heard me come in and greeted me on the landing.

Giddy with joy, I dropped the heavy medical textbooks to the floor and twirled her around. "Mom, I did great!"

When I stopped, she rested her head on my shoulder and hugged me to her. "I knew you could do it," she said. "I'm so proud of you." She smiled. But there was a guarded expression in her eyes, and suddenly terror struck my heart.

"You got the biopsy report," I said.

"Yes."

"Is everything all right? When did you hear? Was it benign?" The questions tumbled out all at once. I tried to read the answers from the expression on her face, but she had steeled herself against this moment, her face a carefully controlled mask.

She didn't answer. Instead, taking firm hold of my hand, she gave it a reassuring squeeze. "Come on inside." She urged me through the doorway, not letting go of my hand until she had closed the door.

Once inside, neither of us sat down. We stood facing each other at the door.

"Mom, is it malignant?"

"Yes." She waited for my questions.

"How do you know?"

"Dr. Karik called Dad at home and Dad called me."

"When?"

"Last week."

"Last week? You've known for a week and didn't tell me?"

"Yes. I told Dr. Karik about the tests you were taking this week, and he understood how much it would mean to you to complete them. So we agreed not to tell you until after your test today."

A sudden fear, worse than anything I had ever experienced, gripped me. "Do I have to have another operation?"

"Yes." Mom's eyes blinked back the tears that kept welling up.

Horrified, I said, "Dr. Karik said that the only surgery left if the cancer recurred would be to have my jaw removed. No! Oh, no!" The cry escaped from somewhere so deep inside that I scarcely recognized it. "And all my teeth and my gums . . ." My hand swept up to touch my cheek. "And the roof of my mouth. Oh, my God, my face, my face. I'll be so ugly."

My mother held me then in her arms, drawing my cheek down to her own. "You'll never be ugly, Bea. And the most important thing is to save your life. You've got to get all the cancer out this time. It's your only chance."

Suddenly I experienced an eerie separation—from Mom, from my dreams, from myself. The voice when it spoke was not my voice. I knew the real me was not inside the body that was about to be mutilated.

"I'll think about it," I said, "but I can't do anything about it for a while. I can't miss school. I have to study for another test Monday. How am I ever going to study with this on my mind?"

"Don't worry about the test on Monday."

"Don't worry about . . . Mom, this is medical school! I can't afford to get behind in my work or I might not catch up."

"Beatrice, you have to go to the hospital on Monday."

"This Monday? Never! I've got to take a test Monday."

"You can't take the test Monday, Bea. You have to be operated on next Tuesday."

"Tuesday!" A dreadful thought came to me. "Mom, what if I have a brain tumor? Did Dr. Karik mention anything about a brain tumor?"

She nodded. "He says he can't tell—that he has to remove all the tissue and bone right up to the base of your skull in order to get the cancer left behind. He just hopes it hasn't invaded the brain."

"Maybe I can get him to put the surgery off until Christmas vacation."

"No, Bea. The surgery can't wait. It must be done Tuesday."

The conversation—my whole life—was now a blur. I could hear Mom reminding me how the deans of MCP had opted to keep me on as a student after my first cancer operation. Now panic set in, dread that another setback might change their minds. But Mom had already talked to Dr. Stanley Fein, associate dean of admissions and student affairs, and quoted his words of encouragement: "We went into this with our eyes open. We had faith in Beatrice then, and we have faith in her now. So tell her not to worry about her studies. When she is ready to study again, we'll send assignments to her at the hospital."

Then we were joined by my father, Donald, who had driven

down from New York, and Mary McFadden, my neighbor across the hall. Mary, a native of Germantown, had worked for the telephone company until her retirement. I first met her that May when I moved in, but in those few months she had become my dearest friend. Every afternoon she had tea and fruit waiting in her apartment when I returned from classes. We chatted about everything, in the way that only trusted friends can. A devout person, she included me in her prayers each morning and evening, and at Sunday mass. It should have helped me to have my parents and my trusted friend with me, but I felt so sorry for myself that I didn't care. I just wished the news would go away.

I telephoned several people from school to let them know of my plight. I was trying to escape, and hoped that someone would offer a solution. MCP statistics professor Dr. George Green was concerned that I might do something foolish in my distraught condition, and offered to let me stay with him and his wife if no one else would be with me. I called Dr. Karik at home and told him how frightened I was. He reassured me, saying it was normal to be scared. And it was calming to talk to a six-year classmate who had known me at Lehigh. She said, matter-of-factly, "You've been through it before. You'll get through it again."

Next I telephoned a classmate with whom I ate lunch every day. He and I had enjoyed one dinner date, and he often walked with me to classes. As soon as I told him the bad news, he said, "Gosh, Bea, that's terrible. I'll come right over."

"No, don't come over," I said. "My parents are here and I have to pack. I just wanted you to know what happened to me because I won't be in school on Monday."

"I'm glad you called me, Bea," he said softly. "I'll call you at the hospital and I'll keep in touch with your parents." His voice sounded concerned in spite of his reassuring words. "Don't worry about anything. You'll be back soon and . . ." His voice broke.

"And what?" I prodded.

"And I'll take you to the class Halloween party." The class Halloween party was to be the second big social event of our class. The first had been a picnic and camp-out where most of us had met one another for the very first time. The Halloween party was to be a costume affair. I hadn't made plans for it, but I really wanted to go to that party. Like any mass of people brought together in a new situation, my classmates had started to separate into social cliques.

Intuitively I felt that I would not be a part of this. I knew that in order to date, to make friends, to become an intimate part of a group during its formation, one must be available, and I wasn't going to be there.

Another classmate rushed over to my apartment as soon as I telephoned her. She and I had first met at class orientation. Ever since then, once a week, we ate dinner together and happily chatted about homework assignments, career goals, and boyfriends. She was slender, tiny, and very vivacious—her buoyant manner now brought cheer into a cheerless situation. "Don't worry about your work, Bea," she said. "I'll offer to help Dean Fein compile homework and notes to send to you."

Early that evening, Sawadh Chitakasem, a teaching assistant (TA) in the chemistry department at Lehigh, arrived from Bethlehem. Chit had been my almost steady boyfriend for two years. During that time he had repeatedly asked me to marry him or to become engaged. Six years older than I, he was anxious to settle down. But even though I loved him, I refused. I knew that such a commitment so early in my studies would seriously impede my progress in medicine. I needed to be free to explore new opportunities, to meet new people, and to make the necessary adjustments to medical school.

As soon as Chit entered my living room, I flung myself into his waiting arms. We kissed and then we kissed again. For one long moment the sweet wild power of his embrace crowded out my anguish. And then I pulled away from him, confronting him face to face. "Do you know what's going to happen to me?" I cried.

"I know." He had steeled himself well for this moment. Keeping his eyes on mine, he reached out and took my hands into his own, guiding me down onto the sofa. And then he sat down beside me, gathering me into his arms again. Still holding on to one of my hands, he reached his other arm around my shoulders and rested his cheek against my own. "Everything will be all right, Bea. You'll see. You've got to get rid of the cancer. That's all that matters."

Even for Chit, I couldn't sit still for long. All that night what bothered me most was the possibility that I might lose my intelligence if I had a brain tumor. I kept pacing the floor, holding my hands to my head and sobbing, "My brain, my beautiful brain." I tried to explain my fears to my parents, to Chit, to Mary. "Can't you see that if I have a brain tumor, I may not be able to think the same after a while? All I've learned will just fade away and I'll never be a doctor. And my face will be all cut up and I'll never be me anymore. And I'll probably die."

Later that night, even though I knew that Mom, Dad, and Chit were sleeping in rooms next to mine, I felt worlds apart from them. Their support made me feel more secure, but memories of how I had suffered after waking from the first surgery loomed great in my mind. I recalled vividly the pain, the choking on blood, the feeling of suffocation. This time the surgery would be more extensive. I prayed that I might have the courage to face whatever lay in store for me.

Early the next morning my mother came into my room. "I waited until I was certain you were up," she said. She eyed the two weekend cases opened upon my bed. I had already filled one with medical textbooks; the other I was still busy packing with toilet articles, extra makeup, and a few of my daintiest nightgowns.

"Mom," I said, my voice barely above a whisper. "I'm so scared." I sat down upon the bed and looked up at her.

She met my gaze directly. "I know," she said, sitting down beside me. "We're *all* scared. Who wouldn't be? But I know that you're going to be all right," she added quickly. "You know how much Dad and I love you. Just remember that you are God's child too and that He will take care of you."

I searched her face for any sign of discouragement, but there was none.

"How long do you think I'll have to stay in the hospital?"

"Dr. Karik told me three to four weeks, depending on how the surgery goes."

"That's what he told me too," I said. "But I told him that I was counting on him to have me back in school by the end of October. And he promised."

"I see." Mom traced her finger over the pattern of my bedspread for a moment. "Dad and I were talking this morning and we agreed that it might be helpful for you to talk with someone else."

"Who else is there?"

"One of the psychiatry professors."

"One of . . . you want me to see a psychiatrist?" I couldn't believe what I was hearing.

Undaunted, Mom continued. "What's wrong with seeing a psychiatrist? That's what they're for, isn't it? To help people with their problems?"

"Mom, I can't see a psychiatrist. I'd be disgraced! I'd be so ashamed!" I stared at her, dumbfounded.

But still she persisted. "What is there to be ashamed of? You have a very real problem. You're not imagining things! And even if you were, why shouldn't you go for help? Isn't that what doctors are for?"

Even though I knew that she was right, I still continued to protest.

My mother got up and walked over to the door. Then she turned her head in my general direction, not looking at me. When she spoke, after a moment, it seemed as though she were speaking to herself. "Why should they think that way? What's wrong with going to a psychiatrist for a little help? I think it's weird not to seek help if you need it." There was decisiveness in her voice as she turned again to me. "If your school didn't respect psychiatrists, it wouldn't teach psychiatry. You must know the name of one of your psychiatry professors." There was no hint of question in her voice. She looked at me directly, locking her gaze into mine.

"Well . . . ," I hesitated. "I enjoy Dr. Stern's lectures, and I'm in his study group. We all have a great time with him. He lets us bring popcorn and fruit and we share it around."

"Good. Call him."

"Now?"

"Now."

"Mom, this is Saturday. I don't have an appointment. He'll be busy."

"Call and ask. Tell him what your problem is. Explain that you are leaving for Long Island and that you would like to speak with him before you go. He just might help you, Bea, and that would be wonderful."

Reluctantly I telephoned the psychiatry department of MCP and left a message for Dr. Stern. Another psychiatrist who was on call agreed to see me immediately. A few minutes later, Dr. Stern returned my call.

"Beatrice! Dr. Stern," he said. "How can I help you?"

"I'm going to have surgery and I wanted to talk with you before I leave for Long Island. I called MCP, but I was told you weren't in. So I made an appointment with the psychiatrist on call."

"She told me about it," he said. "I'm not on call this weekend, but come on over to my home after you see her." He gave me directions.

While my parents and Chit waited in the car, I had a very intense session with the first psychiatrist. She was concerned and sympathetic but soon realized that she was not striking a responsive chord in me. Her own sense of futility and despair at my plight were immediately apparent to me, and she was relieved when I told her that I would be going next to speak with one of her colleagues, Dr. Frederick Stern. She walked me to her door and stood in the open doorway waving good-bye to us.

Dad was the first to speak as he drove us away. "How did it go, Bea? Was she able to help you?"

"Not really." I felt too stunned to speak.

"What did she say to you?" Chit asked. He reached over to hold my hand tightly in his own.

I didn't answer.

"Bea, you were in there a long time," my father prodded gently. I could see the lines of strain etching his face.

"She must have said *some*thing to help you," my mother persisted.

Somehow I willed myself to be objective enough to speak. "She tried," I said. "She really tried, but she was shaken by the thought of this operation. What can one say to a young girl who's going to have a good portion of her face removed?" I never felt more alone, beyond help.

Undaunted, my mother said, "Dr. Stern will think of something."

Dr. Stern's home was in a nearby beautiful suburb of Philadelphia. Again, my parents and Chit waited in the car.

Dr. Stern encouraged me to tell him anything about my life that came into my mind. In addition to my life's story, I told him how I still mourned the death of my cousin Beth, six months younger than I. Beth had died under tragic circumstances several days after her sixteenth birthday. And then I spoke to him of fears about my own death and disfigurement.

At the end of his session with me, which lasted more than an hour, Dr. Stern went outside with me to greet my parents and Chit. It took only a few moments for him to talk all of us into coming inside to have a cup of tea with him.

First he gave us a friendly tour through part of his house. Then he settled us comfortably about his living room and served tea, fresh apple cider, and homemade buns. All the while, he chatted about his family and showed pictures to us of vacation spots that he had enjoyed. He didn't talk much about my pending operation except to say that it wouldn't be easy for me and that he understood my fears. As we said good-bye, he told all of us to have courage and said that he would look forward to the day when I would get back to school.

Next we drove Chit to the bus depot for his return trip to Lehigh. On the way we talked about how much Dr. Stern had cheered us with his homespun manner and about how welcome he had made each of us feel. At school he seemed to be such a formal person. Today it had been a delightful surprise to see him prepare and serve tea to us in an easy, good-natured manner.

"What did Dr. Stern do or say that helped you the most?" Chit asked.

"He told me that my fear is normal—that he, too, would have been terrified," I replied.

It wasn't easy saying good-bye to Chit. We sat together in the back of the car. He held my hand all the way to the bus depot, cradling my head upon his shoulder. "Everything will turn out all right, Bea. Don't worry." His voice was a soft crooning in my ear.

"But I won't be pretty anymore."

"You'll still be pretty."

"How can I be pretty without a jaw? Do you realize what they're going to do to me? They're going to cut off my jaw!"

He reassured me over and over again. "Don't worry, Bea. You have a fine doctor. This time they will get all of the cancer out."

"And half of my head too." A new wave of panic hit me. "Chit, I can't even imagine what I'll look like. They're going to take my teeth and my gums too. Do you realize that?"

"A lot of people have false teeth, Bea. It's not so bad." His voice gentled. "I have a partial upper plate and you still love me."

"We're not talking about the same thing," I told him. "You had your teeth knocked out when you played rugby in Thailand. Sure, other people go to a dentist and get their teeth pulled out, but they still have their gums. I won't have my gums anymore. They're going to saw them right out of my head. You won't even want to look at me anymore."

"How do you know that?"

"I just know it, that's all."

"Don't talk foolish, Bea. I'll always want to look at you."

"Promise that you will visit me at the hospital."

"I promise."

"Nothing will keep you away?"

"Nothing." He smiled at me now, his brown eyes twinkling mischievously. "Wild horses couldn't keep me away."

"When will you come?"

"Tuesday. I'll be there before you're out of surgery." He reached his hand into his pocket. "I want to give you something, Bea."

"What is it?"

"A medal." He held it out to me. "The Miraculous Medal. It will keep you safe. My mother had it blessed for me by Sisters in Thailand just before I left for this new country. I promised her that I would wear it always."

Deeply touched, I said, "I can't take this from you, Chit. Your mother wanted you to have it."

"She won't mind, Bea," he said simply. "She'd be happy to help you. You can give it back to me when you are well again."

My eyes misted with tears as he pinned the medal onto my dress. Then our eyes met, and he smiled. Wordlessly, he cupped his hand under my chin and raised my face to his own. And then he bent slowly and covered my lips with his. I knew then how much he wanted to believe that nothing would change between us. I wanted to believe it too. But deep inside me, a sense of foreboding would not go away.

Several times as we drove away, I turned my head and looked back at his waiting bus. How I longed to go back to Lehigh with him and to shelter myself among the beautiful rolling hills of Bethlehem.

There was just one more thing to be done before my parents

and I could leave Philadelphia for the long drive home to Massapequa. I had to return to my apartment, say good-bye to Mary, and pick up my rottweiler, Sabrina, whom my parents had bought for me soon after I moved to Philadelphia.

"I'll be praying for you, Beatrice," Mary assured me. "And I'll keep in touch with your parents." She wrapped her arms around me, holding me close. I felt the gentle patting of her hand upon my back. "Don't worry, Bea. You'll be coming back to us soon and you'll be all right."

It was late afternoon when we finally turned in to Nassau Shores, Massapequa, a tiny, picturesque peninsula leading into the Great South Bay of Long Island.

"Drive slower, Dad," I said. I wanted to savor every bend in the road, every familiar tree. Our brown cedar-shingled colonial split home nestled in the middle of the street. The street overlooked a deep canal and the bay. Weeping willows lined the curb and danced yellow-green branches in the constant sea breeze. As Dad turned in to our street, I saw our neighbors' cabin cruisers. They pulled against their wooden moorings with every ripple of the gentle tide. I opened the car window and breathed deeply the crisp salt air. From an occasional chimney swirled the spicy odor of oak logs burning. A herring gull trumpeted somewhere over the canal. And then I was home.

My brother, Don, came out of the house to greet us as soon as our car pulled in to the driveway. Handsome by any standards, he was tall and lean with almost classic features and with an immediately perceptible vibrant personality. He was five years older than I, and I had grown up thinking that he always had a solution to every problem that had ever confronted him. Now, as he went through his usual polite motions—greeting our parents, opening the car door for me, helping me out of the car—I wondered what he would say to me.

And then the moment was upon us. He put his arms about me, drawing me close for several seconds before he released me to kiss me firmly on the cheek. "Hi, Bea," he said. "Welcome home."

I reached out to him, and once again we held each other close. And then we walked together, hand in hand, without words, toward the house. Shyly I broke the silence. "Do you know . . ."

He nodded. "Dad told me last week."

I stared at him wide-eyed, my mind whirling like a dervish. If he had known this terrible news for a week, there might just be a chance that he had found a solution. "What should I do, Donnie?"

He turned to stare at me for one quicksilver moment. The set of his face startled me. Instinctively I knew that he was shutting me out, steeling himself against his helplessness. His voice was cool and even. "What do you mean, what should you do?"

"Should I have the operation?"

"Or . . . ?" He waited for my answer as one would wait for the answer of a small child.

"Or not have the operation and just continue as I am and go on back to school." Even as I spoke I knew how foolish I must sound, but I was too desperate to care.

"Don't be foolish, Bea." His voice was grim. "You have to have the operation or you'll die. That doesn't leave you much choice, does it?"

"I could go back to school and go on as I am," I persisted. "I wouldn't die right away and I'd still have my jaw and I wouldn't be ugly."

"Bea, you know better than that," he said firmly. "Go have the operation. There's nothing else to do."

"But if I have a brain tumor, I won't be me anymore and I won't be a doctor."

"You'll be a doctor, Bea." His eyes softened and he turned away from me. "And you won't be ugly."

Inside the house, Aunt Addie, my eighty-six-year-old godmother, and our dog, Speckles, waited for me in the foyer.

"Hello, dear." Aunt Addie's voice rang clear and firm. She smiled and held out her arms to me.

"Aunt Addie!" I wrapped my arms about her and rested my cheek upon the top of her head with its little white cloud puffs of curl. The delicate fragrance of Yardley's April Violets surrounded us. "You smell so good," I said.

Delighted, she gave a throaty little chuckle. "Welcome home, dear," she said warmly.

After dinner, Aunt Addie excused herself. "I'll be in my room, Bea, dear," she told me. "Stop in if you want to have a little chat."

Retired as the principal of Northport High School, Aunt Addie had popularized guidance counseling throughout the public school system and had been a loving guide to my mother through most of Mom's school years. In spite of the difference in their ages, Mom and Aunt Addie had become best friends.

And so it was that my parents had chosen Aunt Addie to be Don's godmother, and later I had adopted her as mine. Through the years that followed, all of us were blessed in the finest sense of a three-generation family.

Now in the gloom of my pending operation, I knew that Don had brought Aunt Addie home from the United Presbyterian Residence so that I could pour out my heart to her in one of our confidential chats. Aunt Addie's body was old, but she kept her mind young and her wits sharpened. And, perhaps, most important of all for me at that time, she was a good listener.

Soon after she had excused herself, I followed her to her room. I spoke to her without any pretense, without any shame. "Aunt Addie," I said, "I'm so afraid. The only thing that I could fear more than this operation would be death. And even death would be a little better than this because death is final, at least in a physical sense, whereas, with this surgery, I'll be changed in some way. I'll have to live with something different." She just held my hand and listened to me as I poured out my anguish.

It is from her that I acquired a technique that I use today with some of my patients. Sometimes there is nothing that can be done to alleviate another's suffering, and at those times, I too have learned to become a listening ear.

Finally, on Sunday, I telephoned Dean Fein. He had given his home telephone number to Mom and suggested that I call him before I left for the hospital.

"I'm afraid," I told him.

"It's normal to be afraid," he said.

"I don't know what I'll do about my studies."

"Don't worry about them. You'll take care of them when you get back."

After we hung up, I realized that he was to be the last contact I would have with my medical school until after my surgery. No more classes, no more professors, no more classmates, and no more friends—just me and the surgery. Everyone had been sympathetic and encouraging, but I realized that no one could change any of the consequences of this operation. I had to go it alone.

# Chapter Two

I TOOK my problem to God. I had been raised in the Lutheran faith, and my family was sincerely religious. They began each day with prayer or Bible reading and prefaced each meal with grace. My whole life I had listened for God's guidance in all my affairs, so I was comfortable turning to Him with the greatest problem I had ever faced. I knew that God would go with me into the operating room. I believed that He would spare me, because He had guided me to the medical profession.

When I was four years old, I woke my parents to tell them that God's voice had come to me in my sleep. He had told me that I would do great healing work, probably in nerve regeneration. "But," I asked, puzzled, "what is nerve regeneration?" The words were not, as yet, in my vocabulary.

Startled out of sleep, my puzzled parents listened thoughtfully. And then my mother explained what she thought nerve regeneration meant. "It must be getting to use an arm or a leg again if you've been sick and unable to use it. Maybe you will help people to do that."

As soon as she could quiet my excitement, Mom walked me back to my room and tried to settle me into bed.

"A crab can grow a new claw," I said. "Why can't people grow a new leg or a new arm if they lose one?"

"I don't know, Bea," Mom said. She kissed me on the forehead. "Go to sleep now. And don't worry. You're just a little girl. When you're old enough to do God's special work, He will make certain that you understand it."

Through the years that followed, I was afflicted with asthma and allergic rhinitis. In fact, at ten I couldn't walk a block without wheezing and frequently missed school. Urine backed up into my kidney, and my ureters had to be stretched. Due to chronic infections and sore throats, my system had been overloaded with antibiotics. This placed an additional strain on my kidneys. Exhausted, I found it impossible to remain awake other than for short periods of time.

By the time I was in the fifth grade, I was absent so much that my teacher sent work home for me. Once she visited to see if she could help me with my studies. Happy to see her, I chatted for a few minutes and then fell sound asleep.

But my mother never allowed me to become discouraged. I was soon to learn the value of small accomplishments. Each day she insisted that we take a walk. I would lean on her arm for support and we would walk the distance of a telephone pole before I had to go back to bed. Then the following day we would walk the same distance, even further if possible. After six months of this, I managed to walk a quarter of a mile. That night we said special prayers of thanks.

Always cheerful and optimistic, Mom reminded me of my goal to become a doctor, and she helped me to keep my dream alive.

"I don't know how you're going to do it, Bea," she said in response to my questioning. "But I know that you will do it. God wants you to become a doctor and He will help you. Remember that."

As a child I played doctor with a toy medical kit and stethoscope. My white toy poodle, lying on a makeshift examining table, was my first patient. While my friends pretended to be nurses and movie actresses, I was always the doctor in the group. Later I recognized the reality of my childhood games— that there is a real need to help overcome the presence of illness and of suffering in the world.

Three times a week, sometimes more often, Mom drove me to Columbia-Presbyterian Babies' Hospital for allergy shots. And during those years I saw medicine practiced at its very best—warm, humane, scientific. My health improved under the care of Dr. Andrew Barrett, chairman of the pediatric allergy department at that time, Dr. Bruce Daving, and Dr. Joseph B. Smith. Those three physicians became like an extended family to me. Over and over again during my many visits to their office, I told them that I too was going to become a doctor. At the end of each marking period I looked forward to showing my report card to them. Year after year I brought in report cards filled with A+'s, and I savored their enthusiastic responses to my happy chatter about extracurricular activities.

Mom encouraged me to explore every talent, to widen my horizons. I took piano, voice, guitar, and art lessons; pursued local political activities; enjoyed writing stories, poems, and songs; collected rocks and stamps; acted; made costume jewelry; and learned to cook. In addition, Mom focused attention on life's true value by instilling in me a deep appreciation of beauty, health, happiness, and public spirit.

Don and I often accompanied our parents to their benefit shows for retarded and injured children. They felt that this would be a good way for us to develop both poise and public spirit. Dad, an executive with NYNEX, the New York area telephone company, was the originator of TELLO, the Telephone Company Clown program, which reached over a million children, filling their lives with laughter as well as motivating them to learn. He also formed the Telephone Pioneer Clown Unit for the Telephone Pioneers of America, Paumanok Chapter. His clown unit was recognized nationally as one of five humanitarian Pioneer themes, and its concept continues to spread to other Telephone Pioneer chapters across the nation.

Mom, a free-lance writer, also entertained youngsters with magic, puppetry, and storytelling. Dressed as Biffy the Clown, Talented Tiger, or Twinkie the Bunny, I sang "The Muffin Man," a children's folk song, helped to make balloon animals, and made chalk-talk pictures, which I gave away. I remember that the garbled speech, clumsy manner of movement, and impaired mentality puzzled me. But the children for whom we performed were so loving and receptive, I realize now that my sensitivity to the needs of the retarded and the impaired stems from that time.

Don was the first person in our family to become a ventriloquist. It all began when he was four years old. He wanted a doll, and Dad said, "Absolutely not." Mom saw nothing wrong with it. But Dad remained adamant. Not one to give up easily, Mom gave it much thought. My brother wanted a doll so badly. Dad felt that a doll might turn Don into a sissy. On the other hand, Mom didn't believe in separating the sexes along rigid lines of activities. And then she had an inspiration. She ordered a Jerry Mahoney ventriloquist dummy and gave it to Don for Christmas.

"This is not really a doll," she told Dad as she wrapped the dummy to place under the tree. "It is a ventriloquist's dummy, and Don can develop a skill from it. Look at Edgar Bergen and Charlie McCarthy."

Still a skeptic, Dad agreed.

As Don grew older, he taught himself ventriloquism from an old volume in Dad's magic library. He thought up innovations and developed a technique of his own. Shortly after he was ten years old, Mom and Dad agreed that Don's skill was now worthy of a professional dummy, handcrafted by a master.

Eventually Don taught me how to ventriloquize. After that, with his help, I developed my first routine with a two-foot-high puppet that I named "Uncle Bunny." And over the years, "Uncle" and I have brought laughter and love to many impaired, retarded, handicapped, and underprivileged children.

Whenever Mom and Dad went on vacation, they took Don and me with them. Often during my preteen years we drove to acreage that we owned on the Lake of the Ozarks in Missouri. Grandma had given this property to Mom. All virgin territory, no building on it, originally it had belonged to my maternal great-grandfather during the Civil War.

It took us two days driving at a leisurely pace to reach the lake. We didn't rush to get there. Like children waiting for Christmas, we savored the anticipation of spending two weeks in the familiar countryside almost as much as actually being there.

And we enjoyed one another's company during the long drive. We have always been a communicating family. Even today we enjoy daily talks and are always sharing ideas. Open and frank, we talk about all manner of things.

Years later, looking back, I realize that this ingrained habit of communication helped me to reach out to everyone about me during my bouts with cancer. There was never any temptation for me to crawl into a shell or to withdraw from life about me.

I realize that everyone needs relaxation and rest, but I like to be full of life, doing lots of things. I don't like to see any day come to an end. But there was something special about night-fall on that lake. In times of stress I often close my eyes, picture that scene, and let the peace that I had found there as a child sweep over me. The early evening sky, sparked with stars, reminded me of the city lights coming on at night. And like the city, the lake had a hustle-bustle, but you had to attune your-self to it in order to be aware of it. In my picture, gravel beaches descend toward the shoreline; fragments of driftwood jut out from the water's edge; cottonwoods cover the land. Various kinds of living things glide and peck and flap, and the reflected light of the moon shimmers as it rides the tide. It's good to form a habit of storing peaceful, beautiful places in one's mind to the memory of which one can retreat in times of stress. Frequently since my surgery I have used this technique to strengthen my inner resources.

Looking back now, I can see that many, perhaps all, of the roots of my strength were planted and nourished in my childhood. As far back as I can remember, my parents had taught me to properly care for the variety of creatures that shared our home and to value life in all of its forms. And I believe that, in order to best defend one's life against a life-threatening illness, one must have respect for life.

I find it equally important to make an effort to understand others in spite of their differences. When one is tolerant of others and is truly able to accept them as they are, it becomes easier to be tolerant of oneself. It was in the first grade of public school, when I was just beginning to learn to read, that I discovered there are different cultures in the world and that learning languages can help to bridge those cultural gaps.

One day a book with a faded brown cover caught my eye. I lifted it down from the bookshelf, opened it, and turned the pages. There were no words that I could read, but the book was filled with pictures of people dressed in strange-looking clothes. And there were pictures of places that didn't seem at all like anything I had ever seen.

My interest piqued, I remained standing at the bookcase, looking at the pictures for such a long time that Mom came downstairs to see what I was doing.

"What book do you have?" Mom asked. I held it out to her, reluctant to part with it. She took it from me, but before she set it back into its place on the shelf, she explained some of the pictures to me. "We won't read this book just yet," she said. "This is written in Spanish. Years from now, you can study it."

With a reluctant glance at the Spanish book, I went with Mom to get my great-grandmother's copy of *Grimm's Household Fairy Tales*. But I determined, one day, to study Spanish.

Today I speak both Spanish and Italian and look forward to the study of as many languages as possible. Already my study of foreign languages and of different cultures has been helpful in my practice of medicine. When non-English-speaking patients come into the hospital, I am better able to help them with their concerns.

My first exposure to foreign cultures came about as a result of my friendship with Mr. Jimmy, manager of a nearby Chinese restaurant. I remember one Saturday before Thanksgiving when Mom, Dad, Don, and my grandfather Poppy, who lived with us, met Mr. Jimmy for the first time. He greeted us with broad smiles and a solid handshake.

"How wonderful to see the grandfather and the parents and the little children together," he said.

Mom, always keenly interested in everyone, asked, "Do *you* have any children or grandchildren?"

"One son, already grown," Mr. Jimmy answered. "But he lives far away, in San Francisco. Chinatown." The words tumbled from him as though they had been dammed up for a long time. "My wife was killed two years ago. Run over by a taxi in Manhattan." He looked at us for a moment, his eyes watery. And then he summoned the waiter and walked away.

Mom and Dad whispered to each other. Dad summoned Mr. Jimmy. "We would like you to share Thanksgiving dinner with us at our home."

"Holidays are very special to us," Mom said. "If you come, we would want you to feel that you are a part of our family."

Mr. Jimmy's face beamed. "Ah, thank you! Thank you so very much! I will be honored to come."

From that day on, Mr. Jimmy became an unofficially adopted member of our family. Although Poppy spoke with a thick Swedish accent, and Mr. Jimmy found it easiest to communicate in Chinese, somehow we all understood one another. And so I learned that a loving heart has a language all its own.

It wasn't until years later, when I too had to triumph over physical handicaps after my own surgery, that I realized what an inspiring example of the human spirit Poppy had set for me. At eighty-five, though growing more frail each year, Poppy worked as a consulting engineer and was a leading authority in floating dry docks.

One evening he said, "Tomorrow I fly to Galveston, Texas— by jet airplane!" He paused to savor the dramatic impact of his statement.

My startled parents exchanged glances. "Whatever for?" Dad asked anxiously. Poppy had never flown on a jet. And now, in his old age, he seldom traveled.

"Whatever for?" Poppy cried triumphantly. "They need me to supervise the dry-docking of the NS *Savannah*. That's whatever for!"

"What's the NS *Savannah*?" Mom asked.

"The NS *Savannah* is the navy's largest atomic cruise ship." Poppy's voice rang with excitement. His faded blue eyes flashed. For a moment he seemed to see the ship. And then he returned his attention to us. "She must go into an old wooden dry dock, and these young fellows don't understand the old wooden dry docks the way that I do." He chuckled. "Imagine! I will be working with the grandsons of the engineers I worked with when I was young."

Within three days, Poppy was home again. Telegrams congratulated him, affirmed his success. For this one last time, Poppy triumphed.

Shortly after that, Poppy's actions slowed. He required longer naps, frequent hospitalizations, and physical assistance. His mental and physical capacities decreased rapidly, and he retired. The plight of the elderly first captured my attention at this time—their loneliness, their physical handicaps, their financial dependence.

Often we found Poppy sitting in the living room with an opened book in his hands. He had always been a speed reader, easily reading two or three books each day in addition to his other activities. Now he never seemed to finish a book. Hours later, after he had first opened the book, he would still be sitting there, trying to read the same page. Time didn't seem to hang heavy on his hands. It just seemed that much of the time he lived in a state of suspension.

I remembered how, as a small child, I had loved to sit by his side while he read. I wanted to show him that I could read quickly also, and I flipped the pages of my book through to the end and said, "I finished." Poppy pretended to believe me and gave me another book to read. Every weekend we had visited toy stores, strolled through the park, and played cards. Now when I asked him to play cards, he obliged, but without interest.

"Poppy's not doing too well," Mom said to me one day. "He needs our help. Let's start our own Ranger Rick club." She groped for the right words. "I'm trying to save his mind. Will you help me?"

After that, every day from five to six o'clock, Mom and Poppy and I held our own version of Ranger Rick meetings. We talked about a wide variety of simple things. At our first meeting, Poppy merely listened. And then, after several meetings, he talked to us, mostly about his father, who had been a noted physician in Jönköping, Sweden.

Years later as I look back upon those meetings with the understanding of a physician, I realize how much those talks had meant to Poppy. They had given him a means of communicating, of still being very much a part of our world. And they helped to remind him that we loved him. That, too, was important. It was a spirit of kindness that I have carried into my practice of medicine.

Eventually Poppy's impairments increased so much that he needed constant care. Unwilling to face the reality of his situation, he tried running away from home. I watched him flee in a taxi, wearing only pajamas under his overcoat. It hurt me deeply to see my once brilliant grandfather, who had spoken nine languages just a few months previous, now reduced to a frail, feeble shell.

That same day, Poppy was placed in a nearby nursing home, where we visited him daily. I remember my mother bringing

Easter baskets to the elderly men—amputees—who were con-
fined to wheelchairs. Tears dribbled down their faces as they
accepted the gifts.

One month later, Poppy died. That was my first encounter
with death. At the funeral home, I sat beside him, trying to
think if there was something I could do, and feeling helpless all
at the same time. Dad knew that I was upset. "Come on, Bea,"
he said. "Let's go get a Coke. There's a deli just down the
street."

The deli was an old-fashioned one with a counter at the back,
where we sat to drink our Cokes.

"Dad, why do people have to die?" I had finally accepted the
fact that Poppy was dead—that he wouldn't get up and walk
out.

Dad looked down at me and his eyes misted. "Bea," he said,
"I don't know the answer, but I will tell you that we will all be
dead someday." Then, seeing the pain registered on my face,
he added kindly, "But remember that time does have a way to
heal all things."

That was the first day that I realized my parents didn't have
all the answers.

Years later, after my surgery, I remembered that day when
Dad had said that time would heal all things. My surgery had
changed almost all aspects of my life, and it had hurt me
deeply. But I had learned that time doesn't *heal* anything. It
ameliorates. It takes away the acute sharpness of pain. Knowing that, I clung to the hope that time would soothe my pain.
And I prayed that the way that would help me to overcome my
hurt would also help me to grow as a person.

## *Childhood Lessons That Later Helped Me to Triumph over Handicaps*

1. Turn to God. Take your problems to Him. Put your
   religious faith to practical use.

2. Respect and value all forms of life. Respect for life can be one of your best defenses against a life-threatening illness.

3. Appreciate the value of small accomplishments. Take one step at a time.

4. Develop the habit of communication. Reach out to everyone about you. A loving heart has a language all its own. Don't withdraw into a shell.

5. Be tolerant of others. Accept others as they are. This will make it easier for you to be tolerant of yourself.

6. Strengthen your inner resources. Form a habit of storing peaceful, beautiful places in your mind which you can retreat to in times of stress.

7. Learn to live in spite of an ongoing problem. Time does not heal anything; it ameliorates.

8. Focus attention on life's true value. Explore every talent. Widen your horizons.

9. Be kind to others. When you bring happiness into the lives of others, your own life will be happy too.

# Chapter Three

MY VISION to become a physician never dimmed. I focused my attention on taking the appropriate courses and participating in activities that would improve my chances of acceptance into medical school. I knew that what I wanted was a highly competitive field, one that would require me to exercise self-discipline and sacrifice.

From talking with physicians I knew that acceptance into medical school would be extremely competitive, that a medical school in the United States might accept approximately one hundred students from a pool of several thousand qualified applicants. And so, even before I had completed the eighth grade, I had mapped out a strategy for my high school years. I wanted to be superbly prepared when I offered myself for medical training, and I determined that I would become the best doctor that it was possible for me to be.

Immediately upon entering the eighth grade at McKenna Junior High School in Massapequa, I went to my guidance counselor and asked to be enrolled in shop. I thought that as a future physician, I should develop my manual skills.

"You can't take shop," she said.

"Why not?" I asked. After seeing the nice things my brother had made five years earlier, I had looked forward to enrolling in the shop class.

"Shop is only open to boys," she informed me.

I appealed to the shop teacher. He remembered having had my brother in his class and recalled what an excellent student Don had been.

"I'd like to be in your class too," I said.

He didn't even consider it. "That's not possible," he said, not unkindly. "School policy. Shop is only for boys."

This discrimination based solely upon sex rankled me. I remembered one summer evening shortly after my third birthday when I had first claimed a birthright of equality for women. Mom had put me to bed. Story time was over, prayers had been said, kisses exchanged, and still I refused to settle down. Mom gathered me up in her arms and carried me over to the window.

"Do you know what we forgot to do?" she asked, trying to put a cap on my restlessness.

"What?" I fixed my eyes on her, completely interested.

"We forgot to say good night to the man in the moon," she said simply. She pointed to a big, round ball of light in the darkening sky. "See the big, beautiful moon up there? Let's wave to him and say, 'Good night, Mr. Moon.' "

I waved. "Good night, Mrs. Moon."

"Mr. Moon," Mom corrected me.

"No, no," I insisted. *"Mrs.* Moon." I waved to her. "Night night, Mrs. Moon."

From that night on, there was no further mention of Mr. Moon. For me, it was always Mrs. Moon who lighted up and kept watch over the night sky. Somehow my child's mind reasoned that where there was a Mr. Moon, surely there was a Mrs. Moon and that she deserved recognition too.

Although disturbed by the injustice of a system that didn't

permit girls to take shop, I didn't allow myself to take it up as an issue. I knew what I had to do. I had to compete successfully in a materialistic world in order to achieve my altruistic goals.

That summer, as soon as I had graduated from McKenna Junior High School, I enrolled in general science at summer school. That fall I was accepted into the biology honors class as a freshman at Berner Senior High School in Massapequa.

High school expanded my horizons. By taking history, science, and language courses, my education encompassed a humanitarian's ideal. It was in some of those classes that I learned valuable lessons that served me well as tools for survival.

At last I got to study Spanish and, eventually, read Galdos's *Dõna Perfecta; Niebla*, by Unamuno; books and stories by Jorges Luis Borges; and Lorca's poems.

Early in my freshman year of high school I wrote an original Spanish poem, "Los Ultimos Momentos de la Vida," which I delivered from memory at Hofstra University during a competition. The poem tells about a dying person who is viewing a storm for the very last time. Others, near him, complain about the storm, but he treasures the thunder and lightning, the billowy clouds, and each raindrop. He knows that he will not experience them again. These are his last link to life before death takes its toll. Today I still agree with the essence of this poem. Many terminal patients have told me that they regret not having appreciated all of the small things of life until their lives are about to end.

All of my high school teachers were excellent, but some had a greater impact upon my future life than others.

Harold Reinhardt was one of these. His European history class brought such ancient periods as the Middle Ages and the Renaissance alive with excitement. My interest kindled, I found myself volunteering to read *Isaac Newton*, by Louis More, during my Christmas vacation. It was a great-sized volume, but Newton's philosophy made a particular impact upon me, especially one statement:

I do not know what I may appear to the world; but to myself
I seem to have been only like a boy playing on the seashore
and diverting myself in now and then finding a smoother
pebble or a prettier shell than ordinary while the great ocean
of truth lay undiscovered before me.

It is reassuring to think that the inquiring mind can never ex-
haust the ocean of undiscovered truth, that challenges will always remain to excite the seeker.

Also through Mr. Reinhardt's guidance, our current world
problems came clearly into focus. Each day he encouraged class
discussion, prodded our minds into action. And he taught us to
view problems from many different perspectives. We learned
to look beyond the obvious. Of equal importance, his students
learned to speak up for issues in which they believed.

Miss Hardin, teacher of advanced placement chemistry, emphasized independent thinking. I was the only girl in the class,
and when the boys grouped together to help one another with
their work, I felt ignored. She never offered sympathy. Instead,
she sternly admonished me. *"You* have to think," she said.
"Don't ask them questions. Have independent thinking." At
the time, her strict manner made that a difficult class for me.
But it was from her that I learned to apply independent thinking to all my science work in college and in medical school.

Mr. Randazzo, teacher of Italian, made each day a happy
one. Although he appeared happy-go-lucky, under this guise
was a very intelligent man who had a rare knack for bringing
out the best in each one of his students. He encouraged me to
accelerate. Under his guidance I read all three books of Dante's
*Divine Comedy* in Italian. Then, that accomplished, he suggested
that I write a scholarly paper about them in Italian. In addition
to learning Italian in his class, I realize now that I was also
learning that no matter how difficult the work to be done, how
great the trial to be endured, each day has a joy of its very own.

My studies continued to go well, and my dream was beginning to shape into a reality. Others began to see this too.

One day as Mom and I sat in Dr. Barrett's office, he held out his hand to me. Laughter danced in his eyes but his manner was serious. "Don't you want to shake hands with me?"

Perplexed, I shook his hand, waiting for him to explain.

"I have been watching you for a long while now," he said seriously. He looked at my mother, obviously including her in what he was about to say. And then he turned again to me. "Congratulations. You have convinced me. You have convinced all of us in this office. You can be whatever you want to be." He turned to Mom. "Claudia," he said, "I'd like to apologize."

"What for?" Mom asked, surprised.

"Do you remember years ago when I accused you of pushing Beatrice too hard?"

Mom nodded. She remembered very well.

I remembered too.

One day, during an office visit, Dr. Barrett had spoken sharply to her. "You're pushing this child too hard," he said severely.

Mom looked puzzled. "I'm not pushing her at all. I . . ."

Dr. Barrett cut her off. "It's one thing to want to do well in school, but it's quite another to burn your candle at both ends," he said severely. "This child is not strong enough for that."

"What do you want me to do?" Mom asked, dumbfounded.

"Don't let her study so hard. Let her bring home something less than A+'s." He glared at Mom.

Mom tried to explain. "Bea's health is the most important thing to me. And I never push her. I never have pushed her. She pushes herself."

"Do you expect me to believe that?" Dr. Barrett snapped. "A young child like this . . ." He turned to me and his voice gentled. "Listen to me," he said. "Do as I say. Don't work so hard and you will feel better."

Now, years later, I heard him saying to Mom, "I'm sorry for the things I said then." He looked at Mom with admiration. "I've gotten to know you and Beatrice very well in all these years. I want you to know that I think you are an outstanding mother. I realize now that Beatrice pushes herself. You don't push her, but you support her in her drive to excel." He blushed and an unfamiliar look of embarrassment came over his face. "It was hard for me to believe at first because she was so young. But . . ." He chose his words carefully. "Beatrice is a very unusual person, very motivated."

Mom smiled. "I'm very glad that you have come to see this for yourself," she said.

From that point on, my allergists shared in my dream.

Dr. Smith, chairman of the Department of Allergies at the Columbia-Presbyterian Medical Center, told me that he had overcome many physical setbacks in order to study medicine. "You can do it too," he said.

Dr. Daving, from the same office, told me that he believed that I could become a doctor or anything else that I wanted to become. "You've got what it takes," he said.

It took self-discipline. But self-discipline was no stranger to me. Mom had instilled it in me from my earliest school years. Each day, as soon as I came home from school, I chatted to her about the school day and about whatever else might be on my mind. After our chat, I took a short nap before completing my homework. My friends knew that I was not permitted to play until my homework was completed.

When Mom had first started this discipline way back in the first grade, I had protested. "The other kids are all out playing."

"You'll join them when you finish your homework," she had said. "First things first."

"First things first" was one of the most valuable lessons that I learned as a child. Because I had learned it well, I had no trouble disciplining myself when I went away to college and on to medical school.

Almost before I knew it, the bicentennial year had gone by and 1977 arrived with the usual fanfare of noisemakers and confetti. As we had done every year since my early teens, Don and I celebrated with our parents at the Shriners' Kismet Temple.

We had good reason to celebrate. The year 1976 had been a great year for our family. Don had made the dean's list; Mom and Dad had completed their year as Worthy Matron and Worthy Patron of their Eastern Star chapter; and I had celebrated my sixteenth birthday. I was a junior in high school, and very much in love with life.

And then, two hours after the new year began, we arrived home. I had just settled warm and snug into bed when the telephone rang. Dad answered it. The next moment, my whole world had been cast into upheaval and one of the dearest parts of my childhood had been annihilated.

Beth was dead! My first cousin, my dearest childhood friend, had died suddenly just before midnight. Four days after her sixteenth birthday.

I loved Beth so much, and yet, I thought, in order to study I had sacrificed time that I could have spent with her. Yet I knew that she would have wanted it that way.

One month every summer and frequent weekends during the year, Beth visited us. Summer vacations that we spent together seemed to be timeless, sun-filled days which followed leisurely one upon the other.

I remembered one summer day when Beth pinned bugs to a cutting board. The bugs were still alive.

"Beth, what's this?" I asked, horrified.

And here she had been so proud! She had caught all these bugs—a wide variety.

She defended herself. "There's nothing wrong with that. They don't feel pain, and I worked hard to collect them."

"I'm going to ask my mother about that," I said. "I think there's something real wrong about that."

"Yeah, what?"

"They're alive."

"This one isn't," she said, pointing to a dead bug.

So I went to Mom as the final judge of everything. Mom told Beth to undo the bugs, but it was too late. Mom told Beth that they had been more beautiful in their natural environment than pinned to a board—that life has value.

Beth looked very sad, but understood. She had worked so hard to prepare this for us. One week later, I asked her if she had done that again.

"No," she said. "I will never do that again."

As she grew, Beth went in fearless pursuit of dangerous activities. She went speeding in her stepfather's car, climbed high on trees that had fragile branches, rode on the back of motorcycles.

I worried about her. "You don't even care about your own life," I told her. "You're going to die one day. You'll find yourself dead."

But although Beth was spooked at the thought of dead people, like so many teenagers she never realized the potential of her own mortality.

She was fourteen on the last summer that she spent with us. She came with Don and me and our parents to watch while we performed on the Joe Franklin Show. One of Joe Franklin's guest stars introduced me: "And this is a new talent starting out. . . ." And then my "Uncle Bunny" puppet and I did our thing. Beth was so proud of us, but my heart ached to see her standing on the sidelines. She had so much talent, but we couldn't direct it properly because we saw her only for short periods of time.

That summer I knew my efforts from then on would have to be directed toward my schoolwork. Summer school subjects took time, and I was doing so well in all of my subjects that it soon became apparent that I would become valedictorian in my senior year if I kept up my grades. This would take time and long hours of study without goofing off. I wanted to soften the blow for Beth. I knew that both of us would be sad not to be together during the summer but that this was the way it had to be.

And so, one day when Mom had driven us to our favorite beach, I complained to Beth of having "no time for anything."

And in her characteristically unselfish, sweet way, Beth said, "Yeah, but you're gonna be a great doctor someday, and you *will* be valedictorian." She was so positive in her wholehearted support of my goal, never jealous, and never begrudging of the increasing time that I had to spend away from her to study.

The following summer I didn't have Beth over to our house. I studied physics all day. But Beth and I talked frequently on the telephone. During one of these talks she asked if we knew any church that she might go to or any minister that she could talk to because she needed some help. We suggested several to her, but for reasons that were personal to her, she didn't approach them.

During that telephone call, she also expressed concern because she had received a grade of C in one of her high school courses. She told me that she had worked very hard in the course and that she really had deserved a B but that the teacher wouldn't listen to her. Years later, remembering this when I teach medical students and physicians, I look beyond their academic performance. I see students not only as recipients of knowledge but also as people with real needs, wants, concerns. This philosophy transcends also into patient care. For the most effective treatment, the physician must consider the patient's entire situation—home, work, psyche.

Beth's death has taught me to be alert to little warning signs that a patient may be undergoing more stress than he or she can cope with. And when I read these signs, I want to be there to lend a helping hand, a listening ear, and a loving heart.

The sharpness of my loss at Beth's death made every waking

moment an agony. There was nowhere in my mind that I could picture a carefree summer again like the kind I had shared with Beth.

After that, I cried a lot of the time and felt all of my goals slipping away from me. My terrible mourning went on for weeks. And then, a few days before a major test in advanced placement chemistry, the teacher's sternness had a special impact on my life. She offered no concern—at least not outwardly—and no sympathy. She said bluntly, "You will have to pull yourself together and go on with your life now or you will destroy your chances of becoming valedictorian. When you are this high up in your class, things are so competitive that you can't afford more than one goof."

Her abrupt, sharp words helped me think clearly again.

"You're gonna be a great doctor someday, and you *will* be valedictorian," Beth had said. I remembered how she had looked that day at the beach with the wind blowing through her hair, and her dark eyes shining. How supportive she had been of me! How willing to sacrifice the time we could have been together! And I didn't want that sacrifice to have been in vain. Once again, I focused my goals.

## *Steps to Shape a Dream*

1. Focus upon your goal. Image it in your mind.
2. Plan your life. Map out a strategy. It helps to know where you are going.
3. Determine to develop your potential. Become the best that you can be.
4. Be willing to sacrifice and work for what you want.
5. Exercise self-discipline. Do first things first as you prepare to meet the competition.
6. Be true to your convictions.
7. See challenges. Expand your horizons.

8. View problems from many different perspectives. Look beyond the obvious.
9. Develop self-confidence. Believe in yourself.
10. Recognize the joy in each day.
11. Inspire others to share your dream.
12. Persevere.

# Chapter Four

Six months later, at the end of my junior year in high school, I ranked number one. For those of us who were college-bound, a special excitement filled the air. It was time to request applications and interviews at the colleges of our choice.

Everything in my life centered around achieving the best possible education for my goals as a future physician. During my senior year I aimed for the highest, presented a good image, persevered through interviews, and learned to laugh at myself. It was during that year that I received guaranteed acceptance into medical school.

Without hesitating, I placed six-year accelerated medical programs at the top of my list. In addition to these, I listed some Ivy League schools. Had I done the right thing to be so selective? I wondered. But shortly I put all doubts out of my mind. *I'm becoming a doctor,* I told myself. *And it's important that I receive the best education possible.* So I wrote to each school and requested an interview.

Dad picked up my pile of letters to be mailed. "You're going to have another busy summer," he said, studying me intently. "Are you certain that's what you want?"

I smiled at him. "Positive. It's going to be very exciting, visiting all of these schools."

"Do you suppose you could find time to let me teach you how to drive?"

"Could I ever! Wow!" I thought Dad, always patient and quiet, would make an ideal teacher. I didn't plan on driving in high school or in college, but I knew that I would be wanting a car in medical school, and this seemed like a good time to learn.

After several lessons, when it seemed that I had a good understanding of the road, we invited Mom to come with us. During the drive, I passed a stop sign without stopping until I reached the corner. Then I cheerfully turned left into the far lane of the intersecting highway, ignoring the lane closest to me. When I finally pulled the car up to our driveway, Mom dashed into the house, dialed the number of the nearest driving school, and enrolled me.

I had enjoyed learning to drive, but the onus of imminent college interviews occupied most of my thoughts. On the one hand, I looked forward to them. I enjoyed meeting new people and seeing firsthand what colleges were really like. On the other hand, just thinking of the importance of the interviews put me into a cold sweat. What if I said the wrong things and blew all of my chances? What could I say or do that would make an interviewer select me above other candidates? How could I convince an interviewer that I was destined to become a doctor?

A few days after Dad mailed my letters to the colleges, I went down to check our mailbox each day.

Mom tried to cheer me. "You've haven't given the colleges time to reply," she said. And then, to get my mind off the interviews, she added, "Dad and I would like to give you your birthday present early this year. How would you like to enroll in Barbizon for the summer?"

"Barbizon?" I was puzzled. "You mean the modeling school?"

"Yes," Mom said.

The thought of going to modeling school intrigued me. Finally I found my voice. "Why would I enroll in Barbizon? I'm not going to be a model. I'm going to be a doctor."

"Dad and I have given this a lot of thought," Mom said. "You've been working very hard, and modeling school would be something completely different for you—a change of pace. We thought you'd enjoy it, but it's only a suggestion. The decision is yours."

"I would enjoy it," I agreed, my initial surprise over. "I'd probably learn all about makeup and hairstyling . . ."

Mom interrupted. "It would help you to make an excellent first impression during your college interviews."

"I don't think so," I said. "My interviews should start any day now, and I haven't even begun Barbizon, so how could it help me?"

"You're supposed to notice improvement immediately," Mom answered. "So even if you've only had one or two sessions before you begin your interviews, what have you got to lose? And besides," she continued cheerfully, "you may not think so now, but there's life after interviewing. Who says that a doctor can't be beautiful?"

It's very important to present a good image to the colleges, I thought. After all, inside my heart I am a well-groomed person with a dedication and a goal; why shouldn't my outer self reflect that? "When can I start?" I asked.

Mom had the answers ready. "This week. The school is a thirty-minute drive from here."

For the next several days I studied Barbizon's brochures. I daydreamed about all the wonderful things that I would learn there, and I decided that the course was a girl's fantasy come true. No question about it! As a Barbizon student, I would walk into my college interviews exuding confidence and poise.

Each class stressed good grooming and cleanliness. Over and over again we were told how important it is *always* to look your best—that you never know who might stop in or what opportunities might come up. Of the many sessions, I enjoyed most the one that taught me how to identify my individual "type." I was told to fill a scrapbook with magazine pictures of models who personified this type. And then I was told to image myself as lovely as these models. I was assured that by the time the course was over, I would have become *as* the person I pictured—that well groomed. Well, I followed the instructions exactly, and with a lot of hard work, I did become what I imaged.

And today, years later, that concept of being well groomed at all times remains with me. Even after a grueling thirty-six-hour on-call schedule as a resident physician, I always manage to be presentable.

Just as expected, shortly after I started the Barbizon course, colleges scheduled me for interviews. I learned a lot from these—not only about the schools but also about myself and about the way decisions are made in the real world.

Some schools, initially high on my list, proved to be bastions of male supremacy.

One interviewer told me that God had gone to his school and that God was a male and that they preferred to keep women out.

Another said, "It's too bad that you're not a man, because we accept only one third women and we want to keep the quota that way."

One interviewer told me that he wasn't happy with women medical applicants. "They're intelligent enough," he said bluntly, "but they're liable to drop out if they get married or pregnant. We've had it happen. It's not right to take a place away from a man who would stay with it." His face was grim, almost accusing as he looked at me.

And so on and on it went. Disheartening, yes. But an eye-opener too. As I threaded my way through the interviews, I found that my anxiety disappeared and I began to realize both the obligations and the responsibilities that a woman aspirant to the professions must assume as an indigenous part of her career. I realized not only that she must be determined to perform to her highest capacity but also that she must be determined to persevere. Her objectives must supersede the personal. Always mindful of those women who would come after her, she must take care that no deliberate action of hers could make their progress more difficult.

Some interviews were especially interesting.

One interviewer asked me to describe myself in one word. I thought, what a funny question! How can a person describe herself in one word? But after a moment, the answer came to me.

"Versatile."

"Why do you say that?"

"Because I'm interested in everything—politics, science, medicine, people, languages, culture. I'm interested in life." The words came tumbling out of me.

At the end of the interview, the interviewer told me that I was a very strong candidate.

But what proves to be a strong point at one school may be considered to be a weak point at another.

After reviewing my transcript and talking with me for close to an hour, another interviewer rejected me on the spot for their six-year medical program. "You don't know what you want," he criticized. "You have too many hobbies, too many interests. I don't believe that you really want to become a doctor."

During a long drive back home, I voiced my concern to my parents. "The medical programs that are interested in me are too sterile. They're too science oriented. That's not what I'm looking for, and the others seem to be too stuffy and stiff."

"Don't worry, Bea, you'll find the right place," Dad comforted me. But I was beginning to doubt.

Mom took me to consult with our friends Doctors Smith and Daving. "Help me," I pleaded. "I'm down to my last medical interviews and everything's going wrong." I filled them in on what had been happening. "I do have many interests," I admitted, "but you know that nothing interests me as much as medicine. I've always wanted to become a doctor."

They nodded, listening.

I continued. "I think maybe my personality comes on too strong, but that's me! If I have to pretend to be something I'm not, then maybe medicine isn't for me."

"Just be yourself, Bea," Dr. Daving said. "You don't need to pretend." He thought for a moment. "But maybe for the interviews, you could tone yourself down just a little." He looked over at Dr. Smith. "What do you think, Joe?"

"Just a little," Dr. Smith agreed. "But not too much. It's important that you be yourself so that they can see how enthusiastic you are."

After the meeting, I felt reassured. I wasn't wrong for medicine. I just hadn't found the school that was right for me. And then I found it in a beautiful setting in Bethlehem, Pennsylvania. And my search was over.

My Lehigh interview was almost a fiasco. Mom and I had just reached Bethlehem and were about to turn in to the campus. In front of us, at the side of the road, the driver of a huge tractor-trailer stood in back of his vehicle, swinging his arms and shouting obscenities. Someone had placed a tiny orange tiger kitten behind the rear wheel of his truck. The driver threatened to squish it. I rushed out of the car to pick up the tiny creature. Just as I gathered the little fellow into my arms, a torrential rain poured down. The kitten, snug and safe inside my cupped hands, purred, but the beige dress carefully selected for this important occasion clung to my body like a wet rag. My carefully coiffed hair had gone haywire. But we drove onto campus, stopping to find a bowl of milk for our poor, emaciated friend.

By the time for my interview, the sun was shining bright and warm. My mother was well groomed, the kitten was comfortable, with a little round belly full of milk, and I was a mess. "How am I ever going to explain this to the interviewer?" I asked.

"Just tell the truth," mother answered cheerfully. "Remember, no matter what happens, you've saved a little creature's life, and that's the most important thing." Grudgingly I agreed with her. It's not easy to be happy about botching up a six-year medical interview.

The interviewer, a Lehigh alumna, gave no hint that it was unusual for her to see a drenched, soggy applicant. With as much dignity as I could muster, I told her the story of the kitten. When I finished, she said grimly, "I hate cats." My heart sank. But at the end of the interview, she smiled. "I may not like cats, but I can see that you are a very kind person and that you have a genuine respect for all living creatures. I'm going to place your application at the top of the list." I named the kitten "Lehigh," and he continued to purr his appreciation all through Lehigh and medical school.

By the time the interview ended, it seemed to me that I had found the program for which I had been searching. My interviewer had expressed approval of my desire to continue history and language studies together with the sciences. In fact, she told me that electives in the humanities were a strong part of the Lehigh–Medical College of Pennsylvania program.

The program, small and selective, accepted approximately fifteen students each year and gave preference to residents of Pennsylvania. The director of admissions, S. H. Black, would carefully evaluate all applications. After that, according to the interviewer, applicants approved by Lehigh would be interviewed by the Medical College of Pennsylvania for final approval. Therefore, although hopeful about my chances of admission, I knew that I must not take anything for granted and that I must continue to be interviewed by other schools.

One week after the Lehigh interview, I was to interview at Cornell University in Ithaca, New York. I told my hairdresser the story of the Lehigh interview, including the kitten, the rainstorm, and my bedraggled hair. "The interviewer was great," I said. "She had a terrific sense of humor, but I can't afford to take another chance like that."

"Of course not," he agreed. "These interviews are important to you. I know that." Suddenly he had an inspiration. He was determined to outdo himself. "Beatrice," he said, "I have been working on a new product for the hair. I was intending to work on it a little longer, but I will let you have it now. It will make your hair come alive. It's a living brew."

He put the product on my hair for a few minutes in order to condition it. Then he shampooed it out, and my hair looked especially lovely. But a short time after I got home, my hair looked like a straw broom, frizz all over my head, standing straight out and dry as could be. The beauty parlor was closed by this time, and we had to leave for Ithaca early the next morning.

"Don't worry, Bea," Mom said. "Leave it to me. I have the solution to your problem." She got out the salad bowl and mixed vitamin E, olive oil, hair conditioner, and raw egg yolk, applied it to my hair, and let it sit for an hour. Then she tried to shampoo it out. Now my hair was not only dry but also sticky.

"Mom, it doesn't look like it's drying."

"Don't worry. That's the oil. It takes a long time to dry."

Time passed and Mom realized that my hair wasn't drying, so she shampooed it again—ten times during that evening. After each shampoo it seemed to look worse than the time before. I should have known that I was in trouble when Mom said, "Go to bed now so at least you have some sleep before your interview. Your hair will be dry by morning."

But the next morning my hair still had a wet, oily look. Mom shampooed it again, and hoping that it would dry during the long drive to Ithaca, we set forth for Cornell.

After two hours on the way, I began to itch, and my hair still looked wet and oily. Mom said, "Maybe we should get it all out." Dad pulled over to the first upstate drugstore that we came to and bought instant shampoo. Mom applied the entire container to my hair right there in the parking lot, but there was no visible change in my appearance. Next, Mom purchased rubbing alcohol. The druggist warned that this might dry my hair too much. Mom replied that nothing could dry it more than it already was and that she had to get rid of some of the grease. She applied alcohol to each strand of my hair, but this didn't work either. After that, Dad telephoned the interviewer, said that we had been unavoidably delayed, and that we would be an hour and a half late. The interviewer agreed to wait for us.

When we arrived at Cornell, Mom told me to tie my hair back and to draw upon the poise that I had learned from Barbizon.

I apologized to the interviewer for being late, and we began talking about different things. I tried my best to forget about my pathetic appearance. But during the middle of the interview, I began to break out in welts. The itching intensified, becoming unbearable. I scratched a little here and a little there, trying not to be too obvious about it. And then I could stand it no longer. I had to get up and move about in an agony of itching, and all the time I was scratching and scratching and scratching. By this time I gave up all hope of getting into Cornell, and thought, *So much for poise and modeling school!* In despair, I explained everything to the interviewer. She laughed so much that tears rolled down her cheeks, and still she continued laughing. I had to laugh, too. It was just so ludicrous.

With me still scratching and both of us laughing, the interviewer placed her arm about my shoulders and walked with me

to greet my parents. She told them that I had a great personality and that I would probably be high on their list of candidates. That April, when the results were in, Cornell accepted
me into their honors program and offered me a scholarship.

My last interview that summer was for the Jefferson Medical
College five-year accelerated program with the Pennsylvania
State University. On the trip home, I complained to my parents
that my mouth hurt and that I didn't feel well.

Mom looked into my mouth with a flashlight. "I've never
seen anything like this before, Bea," she said, her voice puzzled. "You have two black lumps on your hard palate."

Within the next few days, I visited my allergist, who told me
to go to my local dentist. The dentist referred me to a local oral
surgeon, Dr. Steven Rossman. Dr. Rossman was away at the
time, but his assistant saw me on August 31, nine days before
my senior year of high school was to begin. He took X rays.
Then he took a needle and drew some fluid from the black
bumps, cut a little tissue, and told me that he would send it for
a biopsy. Prior to my visit with him, as part of my orthodontic
treatment, I had been wearing a rubber retainer at night while
I slept. He thought that this rubber appliance might have irritated my palate and told me to discontinue wearing it. He also
told me to keep my mouth really clean in case it was a hygienic
problem.

The following week I returned to him to have my stitches
removed, but my tissues had not healed, so I was told to return
one week later. On my next visit, the stitches were removed.
The biopsy report was negative. After that, when I returned to
their office complaining of constant pain and discomfort, Dr.
Rossman told me that my mouth was all right, that I should
take aspirin if I had to take something for pain, and that I
should go to school, concentrate on my studies, and forget
about it. The constant pain and discomfort marred a great deal
of my senior year, but I determined to keep on going in spite
of it.

The *Newsday* Fall Book and Author Luncheon held at the Huntington Town House on October 18, 1977, was one of the highlights of my senior year. Irwin Shaw and Lillian Carter were among the honored guests. Irwin Shaw said that he was looking forward to flying back to his villa in Switzerland in order to write in peace and quiet. I thought, *How wonderful it must be to fly here and there at will!* And then I thought, *Beatrice, you can do anything you want if you really want it enough.*

I had attended the luncheon because I was the co–editor in chief of the *Berner Beacon*, which had been selected as the outstanding high school newspaper in Nassau County during my junior and senior years.

Working on the *Berner Beacon* helped me to develop my leadership ability and to take the initiative in contacts with others. Today, as a resident at Kings County Hospital in Brooklyn, I apply these same communication skills. I talk to my patients and I listen to them and I like to find out what is going on in their minds.

I took a lot of advanced placement courses in my senior year, and one of these was advanced placement biology. The teacher, Anne Brown, was a dynamo of energy and talent, interested in research projects. One day, chatting with her after class, I mentioned my pet herring gull, whom Don had rescued three years earlier when she had been an injured chick. I told her that we had obtained special federal and state permits for her when it became obvious that she would never return to the wild.

Instantly Miss Brown fired nonstop questions at me, and my answers interested her. "Write a research paper," she said enthusiastically. "Submit it to the Long Island Science Congress. I'm working with some of the other students and I will be happy to work with you too." And so I wrote my first research paper, "The Significance of the Oblique-cum-Long Call of 3-Year Juvenile Larus Argentatus as Influenced by Domestic and Natural Environments."

The oblique-cum-long call is the herring gull's trumpet call.

In the wild, the call is made for agonistic purposes, such as when a male seeks a mate, or when the same male wants to discourage other males from trespassing on his territory. But my pet gull uses the call for social purposes, such as to greet Mom or me or to respond when we call to her. She won't give the call to anyone other than us. And even though I have lived away from home for nine years, she remembers me and trumpets a greeting when I come home. The project received top honors.

Although I enjoyed working on this particular project, I knew that I did not care for the isolated life of the researcher.

And then, one day, I received notice that the Medical College of Pennsylvania wanted to interview me. Mom went with me, and when we arrived at MCP, we stood together at the top of the hill, looking at the buildings and enjoying the bright sunshine of the day and the crisp, clean air. Everything seemed so right about the place. A sense of peace and happiness filled both of us, and we felt that this was where I was meant to study medicine. There was no doubt in our minds. "Now all you have to do is get accepted, Bea," Mom said.

I had two interviewers, both women medical doctors. They were pleasant and homey, and I immediately liked both of them. One interview was brief, mostly about financial planning for medical education. The second interviewer said, "This interview will be short. You're young." She smiled. "How much can you have to talk about?"

But that turned out to be the longest interview I had. I was happy about that because I wanted to prove to her that even though I was young, I had led an active, interesting life. During the interview, the interviewer asked a question that I will always remember: "What would you do if you were alone in a cabin in the middle of the woods? There are no people anywhere near you. You have no telephone, no radio, no TV, no animals. You can't go outdoors because there is deep snow all around you. You are completely isolated, cut off from the rest of the world. What would you do to keep from being too lonely? How would you avoid becoming depressed?"

I thought for a moment. "Does the cabin have windows?" She seemed surprised. "Yes."

"Do the windows have any drapes?"

"Yes."

"Well," I said, "I would make a puppet out of the drapes and I would do my ventriloquism and entertain myself." She seemed pleased with my answer.

At the time I thought that it was an unusual question. But in retrospect, I realize that it was a very good question and that my answer to it had been important to her in her evaluation of me. Many times as a doctor, when you are working in the hospital, you are faced with life crises. You are alone when you face them. You have God with you all of the time, but you are alone as far as people are concerned. And in much of medicine you are alone. Even when you face death you are alone. There is a certain sense of loneliness about medicine, and it is very important to know how one will manage to cope with it.

Mom and I left the Medical College of Pennsylvania that day without knowing whether or not I would be accepted, but we loved that school so much that we refused to entertain any negative thoughts.

At the very end of senior year I found out that I was valedictorian. At graduation, the commencement exercise booklet listed many awards that I had received, and I had been accepted by most of the schools to which I had applied, but the Lehigh–Medical College of Pennsylvania program was my first choice, and I have never regretted it. I liked the emphasis Lehigh places on the humanities so that students graduate with a broad view of the world's problems.

On April 12, 1978, I had received the following notification from the Medical College of Pennsylvania:

The Admissions Committee of the Medical College of Pennsylvania is pleased to inform you of your acceptance to the combined B.A./M.D. program with Lehigh University.

Mom and I had opened the envelope together. We held hands and jumped up and down for joy. Now we knew that I would be a doctor and that I had been accepted into my very first choice. We believed that it was a miracle come true.

## More Steps to Reach Your Goal

1. Aim for the highest. Get the best education and training available.
2. Present a good image. Always look your best.
3. Persevere. Hang in there. Be mindful of the example you set for others and of the implications of your actions.
4. Image the type of person you want to become. Fill a scrapbook with magazine pictures that depict what you want to be. Then work hard to become what you image.
5. Assume any special obligations and responsibilities required of you.
6. Be willing to laugh at yourself. Develop a sense of humor.

# Chapter Five

FRIDAY, AUGUST 25, 1978, my first night at Lehigh. Sleep did not come easily. Long after I went to bed, I lay there in the moonlight and peered about my room. That afternoon my parents had helped me unpack. Behind my closet door, I envisioned my clothes hung neatly, my shoes laid out in perfect order. Across the room, my absent roommate's empty bookshelves and bare mattress caught my eye. I'd never met her. She wouldn't be in school the first week, but I wished she could have been there with me. Some kind of virus had gotten hold of her, and I hoped that she'd get rid of it in time for the first week of classes.

All day I had been meeting fellow residents of my dorm. Freshmen like myself, they came into my room, invited me into theirs. They seemed to be a friendly, outgoing bunch of kids. But now that the laughter and the noise of unpacking cardboard boxes had stopped, it seemed almost too quiet. As far as I could tell, the other occupants of the dorm had settled in, and now they slept. But I wished that they'd all wake up and that we could get on with the business of orientation. And then I fell asleep.

There is no gradual acceleration to the pace of campus life at Lehigh. Six o'clock the next morning, the throbbing beat of the Bee Gees' "Saturday Night Fever" started my day. At first, my reaction was one of disbelief, and then I remembered where I was. I got up, opened my door a crack, and gave a quick look into the hallway. Stereos played from several of the rooms. Girls in different stages of undress were finding their way to and from the showers.

A short time later, I walked into the University Center, and orientation began. There were picnics, parties, rap sessions, ice cream bashes, meetings with advisers. And then a grand freshmen and alumni rally at which our class of '82 was "adopted" by the class of '32.

Pilgrimages up the hill to the frat houses started early in the semester and continued all through the year. That was *the* thing to do, especially on weekends. Beer in big kegs, loud music, dancing. Frat brothers wearing jeans and plaid flannel shirts. Freshman girls wearing jeans or corduroys, hair softly curled. Impromptu popcorn and pizza parties in the dorms, movies, concerts, football games. Pranks too! Guys sprayed shaving cream under our doorsills, mooned us as we walked across the campus at night, pinned our doors to lock us in until they laughingly set us free. On and on it went, an endless round of activities charging the campus with sparkling vitality.

At first it seemed as though this free-spirited living was at loggerheads with a demanding academic schedule. But before the end of the first semester, aided by the many university facilities, an understanding faculty, and live-in freshman counselors, such as Gryphons, most of us had learned how to settle all activities into their appropriate priorities. At my dorm, Stoughton House, Centennial II Complex, our Gryphon often invited us for homey chats, especially during the first semester.

I had determined to make a quick and easy adjustment to college life. But things didn't work out that way, probably for several reasons.

First, the constant pain in my mouth. Before I left for school, Dr. Rossman had told me to contact his office only if the pain became worse, otherwise not to worry about it. And so I determined to bear with it, but as anyone knows who suffers chronic pain, it can take a lot of zest out of living.

Second, on the basis of my performance on the College Board advanced placement tests, I had been granted twenty-three semester hours of credit in a variety of subjects. These included Chemistry 21, Introduction to Chemical Principles; Chemical Principles Laboratory; Biology 21, Principles of Biology; Introduction to Biology Laboratory; History 9, Formation of American Society; History 10, American Society in the Industrial Era; and advanced Spanish. This meant that I was taking advanced courses during my first semester as a freshman. Although I had been well prepared, my course work was more difficult than any I had experienced before. In order to grasp it, I had to restructure my thinking and learn to approach things from a more science-oriented base.

Third, I was away from my home setting, and for the first time in my life, I found myself having to cope with many distractions while I was trying to study.

With the exception of my illness, these adjustments were simply a matter of development and were to be expected. They involved a certain maturing process, anticipated by a wise administration. And then suddenly, without being aware of exactly when it happened, I became totally at ease in my surroundings. I became a part of the constant activities and the studies and the laughter. My mouth still pained me, but I was able to rise above the pain and eagerly participate in the full campus life. In short, I had adjusted.

Two of my best friendships at Lehigh were made early that first semester of my freshman year. Both were with professors. I had been walking about, becoming acquainted with all the different areas on campus, when I chanced by the office of Dr. J. Morgan Leslie. The door was open, and a slender, middle-aged man with a scholarly face and patrician features sat at his desk, writing. He glanced up when I looked in. "Can I help you?" A studious reserve etched his face. Clearly I had interrupted his work, and he was anxious to get back to it.

Briefly I explained that I was giving myself a personal tour about the campus. "Are you a professor?" I asked curiously. Other than in an occasional movie, I had never seen a professor actually at work in his own private office.

"I teach history," he replied modestly. "History of Medicine, History of Public Health, The Negro in America."

My face lighted up. "Maybe I'll be in one of your classes then. I'm in the six-year medical program."

Now it was his turn to become interested. "Hahnemann or MCP?"

"MCP."

He put his work aside. "Tell me about yourself," he suggested.

We chatted for the next twenty minutes, finding a common bond in our mutual love of history. I liked him immediately. I liked his gentle manner, his enthusiasm for his subject, and his genuine concern for medical ethics. I promised myself to select one of his courses as an elective in my second year.

When I finally had Dr. Leslie as a professor during my sophomore year, it was a delight to attend his classes. It was obvious that he was interested in his students as individuals and that he felt a deep sense of responsibility to create in each of us an enthusiasm for his course. He brought together the different elements of medical history and blended them into beautiful word pictures, like an artist with his palette. He encouraged students to write extra papers and then shared his free time to discuss these with them. As I got to know him better, I learned that he suffered from severe rheumatoid arthritis, and I respected him because he worked and gave of himself in spite of his handicap. He was a quiet, sweet man, and I grew to love him a lot.

In the first months of fall, the leaves and hills of Bethlehem presented a picture of sepia and shades of brown, unlike the vibrant reds and yellows of autumn that I remembered from home, and the air crisped with the clear, cool days of a mountain town. The grounds were so picturesque that I would take long walks and sometimes at night sit with a classmate on a high hill overlooking Lehigh Valley in order to gaze at the furnace lights of the Bethlehem Steel Mill. It seemed as though we were wrapped in a cocoon of stars. How I loved to walk about the Lehigh campus then! Often Dr. Samuel McFarland walked with me from one building to another on his way from class. He taught Analytic Geometry and Calculus I & II and was my professor for two semesters in my freshman year. A great bear of a man with a shock of iron gray hair, strong features, and snappy brown eyes, he had a hearty laugh that belied his sensitivity. Totally lacking in prejudices and snobbery, he reached out to help any student when he discerned a need, and he delighted in discussing his subject either during or after classes.

At first when I walked with him, we talked about math. But soon our talks became less formal and I got to know the man as he really is. Together we built the nucleus of a friendship, which has continued to grow through the years. I found him to be delightfully human, taking pleasure in the antics of a squirrel, becoming interested in all the tales I told him about my pet seagull, Jonathan, sympathizing with my efforts to survive the organic chemistry course. In short, he was a sounding board for all of my campus life.

I enjoyed organic chemistry, but at times I found it infuriating. I wanted answers quickly. Organic chemistry doesn't work that way. And so I learned to be patient, painstaking, and persistent—good preparation for medical school!

Dr. Richard F. Jones oriented us to the course. He was tall, slender, and clean-cut; little flecks of gray surfaced about his light brown hair. Deliberate and direct when he spoke, it became immediately apparent that he was a strict, no-nonsense professor. When he told us that the work would be difficult and that he expected us to put our noses to the grindstone, we believed him.

At the close of that first class, I was intrigued with the course; a little scared too. And then I recalled the challenges that I had met in my high school chemistry class. *I can do it*, I thought, encouraged.

During the days that followed, I read the textbook assignments and studied diligently. But when I sat for my first test, I did poorly. Here I thought that I had understood everything! For the first time in my life, I found course material that I couldn't quite grasp. But I stayed with it and managed to pass. So much for quantitative chemistry, the first semester of organic!

During the second semester, I studied qualitative chemistry and fared much better. But during this course, I worked on an unknown element for five weeks before I was able to identify it!

During my struggles with organic chemistry, first semester, I made two of my closest student friends: Maria Velesquez and Sawadh Chitakasem, a teaching assistant.

Maria and I became instant friends. I thought she was beautiful with her thick, curly, dark chestnut hair and large, expressive brown eyes. She was friendly, but at the same time a private kind of person, the kind you could trust with confidences.

Our class was so large that we were separated into two rooms about the size of a mini-auditorium for lab work, but we all went to the same big lecture hall. Each lab room was separated into aisles where the students had sinks and Bunsen burners. Maria and I must have been the slowest students in the chemistry labs. We worked in separate rooms, but whichever one of us finished first would wait for the other to come out of her lab.

One afternoon when Maria was still fussing around trying to complete her lab work, I finished my work early and went directly to her room. As usual, "Chit," Maria's TA, was there checking desks. He was required to wait for her to finish before he could lock up. He glanced over at me and smiled. "Hello," he said pleasantly. He nodded toward Maria. "She's really late today."

"That's okay," I said. "I'll wait." I set my lab notebook on the nearest desk and dropped into a chair. "You have an accent," I said, not unkindly. I studied his face. "Where are you from?"

"Thailand." He walked over to me so that we could talk without disturbing Maria. At first I thought he was going to sit next to me, but he continued to stand, leaning back against the wall, hands in his pockets.

I looked up at him with admiration. "You're really far away from home."

"Yes," he agreed. He avoided my eyes. It was evident that something bothered him. Suddenly he blurted out, "Why do you say I have an accent?"

I looked at him, startled. "Because you have," I said. His mouth hardened into a thin line, and a flush crept across his face. "I didn't mean to make you angry," I said. "I like your accent. I meant it as a compliment."

He shot a quick look at me. As we made eye contact, his anger melted. He turned away from me, inhaled deeply, puffed out his cheeks, and blew the air out slowly. Then he turned back to me. "I'm not angry." He spoke carefully, weighing his words. "It's just that you Americans think that you are the only ones who speak English. I have always spoken English. We have some excellent private schools in Bankok." His voice held a tinge of pride. "In fact, our school system is every bit as good as your American one."

"That's very interesting," I said. "I'd really like to know more about your country. I love to study foreign cultures and foreign languages. I just got back from a trip to Spain, and it was wonderful! Flamenco dancers, red-tiled roofs, beautiful sunflowers just like a van Gogh painting!" Interested, I continued. "Do you speak any foreign languages? I speak Spanish and Italian."

"Thai. My mother is Balinese and my father is Thai." His smile grew warm.

I smiled back. By this time I thought he was sort of a nice guy. He was just a trifle shorter than I, but I liked the look of his lean, strong arms and his trim, lithe body.

After that, Chit and I looked forward to meeting and talking after school. We always had so much to talk about. Most of our conversations centered about his brothers and his family back in Thailand, about his desire to earn his doctorate in chemistry, and about the sacrifice that his family had made in order for him to come to this country. I listened enthralled while he talked about Thailand. It seemed so far away, so mysterious. The elephants working in teak forests, the ceremonial dancers, the mountains with their beautiful vistas and waterfalls, the rice plantations. And we talked about my family too—about what it was like to grow up in America.

Poor Chit! He was so dreadfully homesick, fretting when letters from his family were overdue. I could really understand how he felt because I missed my nuclear family too. I telephoned my parents every evening, and at least once every two weeks I received a letter from Don. He had been accepted into a Ph.D. program at the State University of New York at Stony Brook.

"I haven't had time to breathe," he wrote in one letter. "Reports, reports and reports about reports have left me exhausted." And then he had a free weekend in October. He rented a car and drove upstate to Lake George. "Absolutely beautiful up there," he had written after he got back. "All the trees have turned color (bright oranges, reds, browns, yellows intermixed with a few struggling greens). I've often wondered why decay (fall foliage) is so beautiful. You'd imagine it to be disgusting and morbid; yet it's quite refreshing. The cabin we [he and his friends from school] rented in the Adirondacks was bathed in these vibrant colors from the overhanging leaves of mountain forests. When we woke up in the morning, we'd watch the sun rise over the mountain peaks and flood the valley with golden yellow and pink fingers which interlaced with the vapory mist rising off Lake George. Splendid—absolutely splendid!" And then he talked about his subjects and signed, "So long, Bea. I love you and will keep you in my prayers. Love, Donnie."

I read the letter to Chit, and he was very impressed with the poetry of it. "Your brother sounds like a great fellow," he said. "I'd like to meet him one day."

Finally Chit invited me to a rock concert on campus. That was our first date. After the concert he walked me back to my dorm. I was surprised that he didn't treat me to a soda or something, but I had a little apple in my purse and I shared that with him. When we reached my door, he invited me to dinner that coming Friday. We agreed to meet at the Mart Science Library. His eyes twinkled as he said, "I'll cook a Thai dish just for you!" Then he bade me a formal good-night.

Friday night I went to meet him in the library.

"Chit isn't here," one of my friends in the six-year program told me. She stared at my portable tape recorder. "Take your recorder over to his office and play it outside his door. He'll come out to see what's going on. He'll see you. That'll jog his memory and then you're in business." She shrugged. "He's just absentminded."

On the way to his office, I played "Summer Love" from *Grease,* and when I reached his door, I turned up the volume loud enough for him to hear it.

He came out, surprised to see me. "What are you doing here?"

I looked annoyed and as unfriendly as I could. "Nothing."

"Nothing?"

"Listening to the music," I tossed off with an air of unconcern.

He stood there, bewildered, uncertain what to say. Clearly he was puzzled by my strange behavior.

There was an awkward silence. Finally I blurted out, "You promised to make dinner for me tonight and you forgot about it. That wasn't very nice, so I don't want to have anything to do with you anymore."

He stared silently at me, taking several seconds for my words to sink in. Then, as he remembered, his brown face paled. "Oh, no!" he said, clasping his hands to his head.

I turned to walk away, but he moved quickly and placed himself in front of me, blocking my exit. "Please, I forgot." He looked directly into my eyes, his face flamed with embarrassment. "I . . . I was thinking about my work . . . my family. My uncle was sick when I left home and I haven't heard anything."

I stiffened and he stepped aside. "Please!" he called after me as I walked away. "I do want to make dinner for you!"

That night I ate dinner at the University Center with one of the guys from my six-year program. Afterward we were joined by some others, and all of us carried on a salt-and-pepper fight like a bunch of wild kids. It was good sport, but I couldn't get Chit out of my mind. I really liked him and had looked forward to sharing that free evening with him.

It was still early when I got back to my dorm. I telephoned Maria. "Beatrice, don't be a fool," she said. "The guy's crazy about you. Call him up."

I phoned him and he answered at the first ring. "I'm really happy you called," he said.

"What would you have done if I hadn't called?"

"I would have called you." We both laughed.

"You're really no good for anything, but I like you anyway," I said cheerfully.

"I'm really sorry about dinner. I'll make it up to you."

"When?"

"How about next Friday?"

"Next Friday! You can wait that long to see me?" I teased him, now that I was certain of his interest.

He chuckled. "Of course not! What are you doing this evening?"

I wondered if he was aware of the music in his voice, the mellow tone of his soft accent. "Well . . . I was supposed to be having dinner with a Thai. . . ."

"I'll be right over."

"How will you get here?" He lived up the mountain at Smaggs, a residence for graduate students, and there wasn't much transportation available in the evening.

"There's a bus. I'll come right down now."

A short time later I had put on a soft woolen maroon skirt and a long-sleeved bone blouse with a background of tiny maroon flowers. I set up my strobe light, got my popcorn maker ready. I didn't have long to wait. He had caught a bus right away.

As soon as he came into my room, the first thing that he noticed was my roommate's stereo. He went absolutely crazy over it. "That's a fine stereo," he said. "It's the best one I've ever seen. May I play it?"

"Sure." My roommate had told me to use it whenever I wished, but I had never used it. I was always glad to have things quiet around me, except at parties.

We danced several dances and then we sat down next to each other on the couch, held hands, and talked. And then he kissed me.

After that we saw each other every day, even if only for a few minutes. And we talked on the telephone every night. But we never allowed our relationship to interfere with study. Sometimes we studied together, but most often we found that we did our best work alone.

On occasion we double-dated with Maria and one of her friends. The weekend of the Lehigh–Lafayette football game, Maria invited us and a small group of our mutual friends for dinner. The campus ran wild with excitement, and we were a wonderful part of it.

For a while things went well, and then one evening in the beginning of November as I walked back to my dorm from the University Center, I felt a sudden, almost unbearable pain coming from deep within the tissues of my palate. I had endured pain constantly ever since my first biopsy in Dr. Rossman's office the year before, but now, in addition to this intense pain, I was having trouble breathing.

As soon as I reached my room, I looked into my mouth. My palatal arch had been effaced with swelling. I had no palatal arch—absolutely none! I ran into my dorm's bathroom and rinsed my mouth, but that didn't help. The swelling increased, partially blocking off my throat. Fear gripped me. I didn't know what to do or whom to go to for help because I had been told that there was nothing wrong with my mouth. But I knew that something was not right. Next, I rinsed my mouth with salt. When that didn't help, I put a little salt under my gums. That hurt dreadfully, but it did make the swelling go down.

Immediately after that, I returned to my room and telephoned Dr. Rossman. I reminded him that he had told me to contact his office if the pain became worse. I told him what had happened and that the pain was now just barely tolerable. He made an appointment to see me at my convenience as soon as I got home during the four-day Thanksgiving weekend. I thought that I could manage to keep on going until then.

I had brought my Bible with me from home and I read it every day, not any special passages, just verses that filled my need as I thumbed through it. It comforted me to feel God's presence. For pain, I took Empirin or aspirin. Chewing had become difficult, so I stopped eating popcorn and ate only soft foods, such as cottage cheese, Jell-O, and liquids.

Because of the pain, it had become more difficult for me to concentrate and it took me longer to complete my studies. Chit knew of my problem, and he was very patient and understanding. Sometimes he would invite me to his apartment at Smaggs, and while I studied, he would fix dinner. His mother sent recipes and he adjusted the amount of spice so that it wouldn't irritate my mouth.

In retrospect, I believe that Chit and I had fallen in love instantly but that neither of us was aware of it until later.

I remember the first time I saw him. I was sitting near Dr. Jones in a little room in the basement of Mudd Building. I wore yellow pants and a yellow polka-dotted shirt and I looked very pretty and I had just come back from Spain and I thought the world was beautiful. Chit bounced in, and then he bounced right out after Dr. Jones introduced him. He reminded me of a deer in the woods—thin, graceful, with enormous brown eyes. He didn't try to make a big show of himself in order to impress anyone. He simply came in and then he left. I thought, *My! How unusual!* After that, even when we were going together, he always reminded me of a deer in the woods. He moved so quickly, so gracefully, as he scampered about. And he was so quiet.

When the first snow fell that autumn, I remembered that he had never seen snow other than in the movies. I wanted to share this experience with him, but we were both busy that day. I pinned a note to his office door. "This is the *real* snow. Enjoy it!"

My parents weren't aware that Chit and I were becoming romantically involved, but whenever I telephoned home and talked about school, I also talked about Chit. Mom and Dad said that they looked forward to meeting him. This wasn't unusual because they had always met all of my friends. So when I packed my bags for the Thanksgiving weekend, I left them in Chit's office at Mudd Building.

Dad picked me up there and met Chit. I was happy to see how well they got along. But my heart ached when I saw Dad. I realized how much I had missed him, and I saw, too, that

some of his hair had gotten white in the short time that I had
been away.

Back home, I kept my appointment with Dr. Rossman. I told
him my palate hurt. It was swollen, and I had trouble chewing
and some trouble breathing. I also told him that the swelling
had gone down after I had applied the salt, and he laughed. At
that time he mentioned that he would want to put me in the
hospital. I asked him if I could wait until Christmas vacation.
He said, "All right." We had a four-week Christmas vacation;
Thanksgiving break was only a long weekend.

My high school boyfriend had come home for the Thanksgiving weekend too. I had received his letter addressed to me
at Lehigh.

> Dearest Lady,
>     This is to inform you that I have not forgotten the woman
> I love. . . . I returned home on Columbus Day only to find
> that the girl I love did not also return. . . . I can't wait to
> see you over the Thanksgiving holiday. And that pie can
> wait [I had promised to bake a pie] until after I'm able to
> put my arms around you and hold you. I live for that
> moment. . . . I hope you're successful at Lehigh and are as
> happy there as I am whenever I think of you. . . . P.S. I'll
> see you as soon as I arrive for Thanksgiving, so be ready to
> see me, beautiful.

He was waiting for me as soon as I arrived home from Dr.
Rossman's office. He was tall—about five feet eleven—with
wavy, dark hair carefully trimmed in order to provide the best
possible frame for his classic features. His well-shaped mouth
sported a neatly trimmed mustache, a wide smile, and even,
white teeth. Everything about him spelled vitality and easy
charm. His long-lashed gray eyes held a hunger that would
have stirred me before I met Chit. I knew that I would have to
tell him the truth. It was the only fair thing to do.

A few minutes later, we were driving to dinner. Suddenly he

pulled his navy sedan over to the side of the road and gathered me into his arms. "At last we're alone," he said. He bent his head down and kissed my lips. Instantly his mouth became possessive, demanding. And then, with a sudden force of will, he released me and leaned back against his door, facing me. "You mean so much to me," he said huskily.

And then I told him about Chit.

His face clouded. When he spoke, his voice was taut, restrained. "Are you telling me we're through?"

"I'm not certain," I said. I wondered how I could be saying this to him. Just a few short months before, we had agreed that I should return his high school ring before I went away. At the time, we both thought that we were being very grown up, removing any visible obstacle to new relationships that we might make at our different schools. But, of course, neither of us had expected this to happen.

He looked down at his hands clenched into tight fists, knuckles whitened from the pressure of his grip. Then he looked up at me. "He's not even American," he said bitterly.

I nodded.

"Think about it, Sandy." He called me by his nickname for me. "You know that I care, but I won't force you. It's up to you."

During dinner we talked about all of the things that had happened to us in the short time that we had been in college. We compared the difficulty of our courses, talked about new friends. I told him about the trouble I had been having with my mouth. He couldn't resist teasing me. "I always knew your mouth would get you into trouble."

He continued to write to me at Lehigh—cheerful, affectionate letters that never mentioned the possible rift in our relationship. And then, two weeks before Christmas, I wrote to him of my decision to continue dating Chit.

He responded with a letter detailing his activities at a fraternity where he had celebrated the receipt of my letter by becoming very drunk.

If I really believed that I had lost you, I would be very
hurt. In fact, I would be tempted to blow up an entire
midwestern city.

During Christmas vacation, he came to my house and rang
the bell. My parents told him that I wasn't home. After that, he
raced past my house on several succeeding holidays, revving
the engine of his sedan, but I never heard from him again.

It was close to Christmas when we had a spaghetti dinner in
my dorm and gathered about a Christmas tree to exchange
small presents. Mine were two star-shaped ornaments of terra-
cotta, which I have hung on our family tree every year since
then. Mom and Don drove over and picked me up at Chit's
apartment. We had exchanged presents that evening, and a
group of us had gathered to celebrate the beginning of the
holidays. Mom and Don joined in the festivities, and Chit,
smiling and gracious, was delighted to see them. Maria was
there too, and Mom liked her at once. When we left, Chit
walked with us to the car. He opened the door for me. As I
started to step inside, he planted a quick kiss on my lips.
"Merry Christmas," he said. "I'll come to see you as soon as I
can." He stood there waving to us as we drove away.

The next morning he telephoned. "I love you," he said in
Thai. The warmth of his voice set my heart on fire. A few days
before the Christmas holidays, Chit had committed himself to
me and had proposed marriage. I had told him that I loved him
but that I couldn't limit myself at that early a stage in my
studies—that I didn't know what demands medical school
would place upon me. He agreed to be patient and not press
me for an answer.

On the twenty-first of December, I went to Dr. Rossman's
office, expecting to be hospitalized. My palatal arch was less
swollen than it had been, but it felt hard and it hurt. I still had
trouble chewing and some trouble breathing. I also had a cold.
Dr. Rossman gave me a prescription for erythromycin and told
me to see him the day after Christmas.

The cold lingered through the holiday season. Chit visited my home and celebrated New Year's Eve with my parents, Don, and me at the Shriners' Kismet Temple. Shortly before midnight, he joined with me in saying a prayer for Beth.

Finally, on January 11, my cold was over, and I asked Dr. Rossman if I could go into the hospital. I still had one week of vacation remaining. He said that wouldn't be possible but that he could hospitalize me in February or in March.

I said, "That won't fit with school vacation. Can it wait until May? That's the end of my freshman year, and there is a break before summer session begins." He said that he thought so.

After my visit to Dr. Rossman that day, I went to Dr. Smith and asked him to telephone Dr. Rossman in order to find out if my mouth condition was serious or if I could safely postpone going into the hospital until May. Dr. Rossman told me that Dr. Smith had called him and that he had told Dr. Smith that there was nothing to worry about—that I could safely postpone going into the hospital until May.

During the ensuing months my palate became harder and more painful. I curtailed nearly all of my social activities and devoted myself to study. Chit was very sympathetic and concerned. But both of us were under a tremendous strain. We looked forward to May, when everything would be fine again.

It snowed often that winter. Sometimes it snowed so heavily that classes would be canceled. Then Chit and I had some of our best times. We made an impromptu holiday—went for walks, had snowball fights, trudged through the snow like two kids. Later we'd go to the movies on campus. I wore purple pants, a purple shirt, and a purple scarf. Chit told me over and over again, "You look so pretty, Bea. So pretty!"

That was my last semester of English, and I enjoyed sleeping late on the weekend, then waking up to read a novel, such as *Wuthering Heights* or *Pride and Prejudice*. Dr. McFarland continued to make analytical geometry and calculus II interesting. Organic chemistry and lab continued to challenge and to fascinate me. Introduction to the Theatre was an easy elective, and

Chinese Civilization was taught by a young-looking middle-aged professor with such a soft, clear voice that it was a joy just to sit and listen to his lectures.

Founder's Day 1979 I received freshman honors from the faculty of Lehigh University in recognition of high scholastic achievement during the academic year 1978–79.

The college year ended in May. Then, after a short break, the six-year medical students would return to continue their studies through the two summer semesters. I sat for the last final of my freshman year on Mother's Day, May 13. The following day I entered Brunswick Hospital. Tuesday, May 15, Dr. Rossman operated on my palate. It was two months and one day before my nineteenth birthday.

My pastor was the first person I saw when I went to the hospital. He met Mom and me downstairs in the waiting room. Mom had asked him to pray for me, and he had volunteered to visit. There was nothing alarming about that. It is the custom in our church to request pastoral and/or congregational prayers both in times of celebration and in times of need. Some of my friends and classmates at Lehigh had promised to pray for me too.

That evening Dr. Rossman came to my room and looked in my mouth with a light. I told him that my mouth hurt a lot, that it seemed to be harder than it had been, and that it was gray. Grasping at straws, I asked, "Do I need to go for surgery?"

"Yes," he said. "Don't worry. It is probably a cyst, but we will go in tomorrow anyway and take it out."

I was frightened, of course. But I was confident that my life would get back to normal after the surgery and that I would finally be free of pain. I expected to be completely healed within two or three days.

I was not awake during the operation. The first thing that I remember was waking up in the recovery room. I couldn't breathe because blood was coming out of my nose and my mouth, and I was choking on it and swallowing it. Each time I went for air, I swallowed more blood and I was scared. I was panicking because I didn't know my nose was full of blood and stuff and I couldn't breathe. I screamed for the nurses. They held me up in the bed because I was vomiting nonstop and choking and suffocating all at the same time.

I remember one of the nurses bending over my bed, trying to help me.

"Is it cancer?" Somehow I managed to get the words out, but I was in a lot of pain.

"I don't know," she said.

They gave me three needles, and I heard one of them say, "Poor girl."

When I returned to my hospital room I still felt smothered and I was in a lot of pain. I couldn't breathe out of my nose, and my mouth felt clogged.

Dr. Rossman didn't mention any diagnosis to me. When I asked him about my condition, he said, "We'll put you on a soft food diet." I asked him again, and he repeated, "I'll put you on a soft food diet." And then he left the room. He never said anything about what he had found in my mouth. I had no idea that I had cancer. When I was discharged from the hospital on May 17, I did not have a diagnosis.

Chit visited for the weekend and went to Dr. Rossman's office with my parents and me on May 18, the day after my discharge.

First Dr. Rossman removed the small stent that he had placed in my mouth immediately following surgery and replaced it with a clean one. The stent was a small prosthesis that Dr. Rossman had made before surgery so that it could be used to cover the hole in the roof of my mouth until that could heal and close. It wasn't a tight seal, and I had to constantly hold a tissue to my nostrils to catch the leakage from whatever I ate or drank. This was embarrassing and uncomfortable, and my mouth was painful. All of this was supposed to be a temporary condition that would heal quickly.

As soon as the stent was in place, Dr. Rossman told me that I had mucoepidermoid cancer and that he was worried. He said that cancer is nothing to toy with and that I wouldn't be able to have children because hormonal changes could take place with pregnancy and might trigger the cancer again. But he said that with no major or hormonal changes, I could be cured forever, that he had gotten everything out, and that I could rest assured that I was cured. But in the meantime, he said that he didn't know if the cancer had spread to my lymph nodes and that he would like to do blood tests and more work on me. Then he asked me if I would go to the Long Island Jewish Head and Neck Conference on May 22.

"Don't worry," he said. "I got three margins. They were clear. But I didn't get a fourth margin." I didn't understand what he meant, but I understood that I had cancer. Years later I was to learn that if a fourth margin had been removed, I could have been spared much of my radical surgery.

Things happened quickly after that. I had CAT scans and tomograms done at North Shore Radiological. That Sunday, May 20, Mom graduated from Adelphi with her B.A. degree. I wanted her to attend, but she wouldn't leave me. I was sad about that but felt too ill to protest.

At the Long Island Jewish conference, no discussion took place in my presence. Those present looked at my mouth, and then I waited outside in the hall until the conference was over. Half an hour later Dr. Rossman introduced me to one of his colleagues, an internist who had been present at the conference. I agreed to visit the internist at his office later that day.

At his office, the internist took a wire with a light on the end, a scope, and looked up my nose. He said that I had irritated tissues or possibly cancer. He couldn't tell, he said, because it was too soon after surgery. And then he made an appointment to see me two weeks later.

On May 25, I returned to Dr. Rossman's office and told him

what the internist had said. Dr. Rossman replied, "Don't worry. It couldn't be cancer. It's just irritation."

"I would like to have a medical doctor follow my case," I said.

He took objection. "You don't need a medical doctor. I can check you, examine you. I will take a little more tissue now, just to check out how everything is." Then he put me to sleep with a general anesthesia in his office.

When I woke up, my mouth was more open than it had been after surgery. There was a little hole at the top of my mouth. It was all cut, bleeding, and very sore. I said, "I didn't know you were removing that much tissue. It looks worse than after surgery."

"It will heal up. It will close," he said. Then he told me that they weren't sure whether or not they had to do another operation on me. They wouldn't do anything just then, he said, because I needed time to heal, that I had been through a lot.

I said, "While they are deciding what to do, I'll go to school. Is it all right to go to school? I have to go back for summer school."

He said, "All right, but don't let them know you had cancer. Don't tell the medical school you had cancer because they might kick you out of your program. They like accelerated students to be healthy. Medical schools don't like people to be sick." I agreed to see him at the end of my first session of summer school, and he scheduled surgery for me at Long Island Jewish for the twelfth or thirteenth of July.

Now I was in a real dilemma—to tell Lehigh or not to tell Lehigh. If I reported my cancer to the university, would they drop me from the six-year medical program? If the university didn't drop me, would the medical school drop me?

To all outward appearances, I was young and healthy. My tumor had been small. According to the hospital laboratory report, they had received a specimen from Dr. Rossman that was 1.5 by 1.8 by 1 centimeter, about the size of a woman's watch, the size of a dime. Dr. Rossman had told me that he had gotten three clear margins and that although he hadn't gotten a fourth, he believed that he had gotten all of the cancer and that I had nothing to worry about. Why, then, should I jeopardize everything I had worked for? The cancer had been cut out. It was no longer a part of my life. Why mention it?

# Chapter Six

AT the beginning of Summer Session I, I moved into a private room in one of the older buildings on campus. My greatest fear was that I might be dropped from my medical program.

The small hole in the roof of my mouth that had been made by the surgery hadn't healed, and much of what I ate and drank spilled out through my nostrils. Exhaustion from the stress of surgery and from the anxiety of not knowing just how much and in what way cancer might continue to plague me took a severe toll, both physically and emotionally. But each day I regained a little more strength.

A few days after my surgery, Mom had telephoned her physician cousin. She thought that he would be well qualified to advise me. Jeff had been Commandant of Bethesda Naval Hospital and Portsmouth Naval Hospital. His answer was immediate.

"Beatrice should tell the Lehigh medical department about her cancer. It's best to have things out in the open right from

the beginning. That way, if she should need to have treatment
in the future, she could expect to have the support of her medical school."

And so as soon as I returned to Lehigh, I reported the results
of my surgery. Mrs. Moss, health professions coordinator, listened without interrupting. Only a faint, barely perceptible
flush about her face betrayed her emotion. Then she reached
into her desk and pulled out a file of papers. "You've been
through a lot," she said. "I'll adjust your course load for the
summer. Take biochemistry this semester. That will be
enough." I realized with relief that she hadn't said, "You have
to drop the program." Instead, she was saying, "Don't worry.
You have enough AP credits to carry you."

"I planned to use those to take advanced courses," I said
sadly, reluctant to give up my plans to excel.

"But now they will serve an even more important function,"
she said gently. "They will keep you current with your peer
group and they will allow you time to recuperate." She smiled
at me. "And if the biochemistry is too much for you, tell me,
and I'll get you out of it."

Long after I left her office, I could hear her voice in my mind,
"Don't worry. We'll work something out." I knew that I had
started college with more advanced placement credits than
most of the students, and now I knew that those credits would
keep me from falling behind.

Each day Chit visited, and Rachel Breslow, one of my six-
year classmates, wrote cheerful letters to me throughout the
summer. I had been a weekend guest at her home the previous
fall, and she had told me then of her love of art. Her talent
amazed me, and I was lavish in my appreciation of her work.
Her eyes had glowed with unconcealed delight as I praised her,
and I knew then that art, not medicine, was her life. Soon after
that, she surprised me with a large picture of a panda rolled up
and tied with red ribbon. "For your birthday," she said.

"This is October. My birthday is in July," I said.

"This is to make you happy in July," she said. How prophetic!

July 5, biochemistry completed, I returned home for the remainder of the summer.

Four days later I went to Robert Karik, M.D., at Columbia-Presbyterian Medical Center for a second opinion. Dr. Karik, a maxillofacial surgeon, oral surgeon, plastic surgeon, dentist, and physician, took my medical history and examined my mouth but explained that he couldn't say much at that time. He hadn't received my records from Dr. Rossman.

The following day I went to Dr. Rossman. I told him that I had seen Dr. Karik, and again I requested that he send my records to him for a second opinion. Then I reached into my purse and took out a little sliver of bone wrapped in tissue.

"What's this?"

"Bone. It worked itself out of my palate when I was at the movies."

Dr. Rossman took it from me and looked at it. "This isn't bone. It might have been popcorn."

I insisted that it was bone.

Dr. Rossman examined it closely. "You're right," he said. "It is bone. Let me keep it." He folded it carefully into the tissue and then he said, "I want to have a look at the bone up there. Let me do that now. Everything might be fine and then you might not need the surgery on the twelfth or thirteenth." He explained that he wanted to take out a little bit of bone from the fourth margin, the margin that he hadn't gotten during the operation. By this time my mouth had started to heal and I didn't want to go through another procedure. But, hoping to avoid being hospitalized, I agreed.

He administered intravenous Valium and put me to sleep. When I woke up, the first person I saw was Mom. I was in a recovery room in Dr. Rossman's office.

"Why is she crying?" Mom asked.

"That's normal," Dr. Rossman answered her. "That anesthesia does that to some people."

My mouth was sore and bleeding. All the healing skin was gone and again it looked the same as it had after surgery. There was a little hole in my palate again. I said, "You never told me you would take out all that tissue. The hole's as big as it was before, and it had just begun to heal."

When I saw Dr. Rossman again, he said that he was positive that he had gotten all the cancer out but that I should see him at the end of August before I returned to Lehigh. When I asked him about the results of the procedure that he had done in his office with the bone, he denied having done it.

"You must remember," my mother said. "You put her to sleep."

Again he denied it. He shook his head. "What procedure? I never did anything like that. I don't know what you're talking about."

Mom and I were puzzled by his denial, but we were happy that his office telephoned to cancel my scheduled surgery at Long Island Jewish Hospital. My first thought was to return to Lehigh for the second summer semester, but then I reconsidered. It would be better to use the remainder of the summer to restore my energy.

This was a difficult time. Terrible doubts nagged us. We had been told that the floor of my nose had been cut into and that it was a possibility that cancer cells had been spilled into the blood.

"Cancer doesn't disappear," Dr. Karik said. "We will just have to wait and see where or if it will appear. If Beatrice were my patient, I would do another biopsy, but I won't do that unless she is in my care."

Before the end of that July, my parents asked Dr. Karik to be my physician. He performed a biopsy of my palate on the twenty-sixth of July at Columbia-Presbyterian, and we were relieved to learn that it was benign. On the fourth of August I had a CAT scan. Immediately after that, Mom and I flew to San Francisco to rest and relax.

It seemed to me now as if I had entered into a state of permanent anxiety. For the first time in my life, I didn't have any idea of what the future held for me. I didn't know whether or not the cancer had spread. I didn't know whether I was going to live or die. When you go on vacation with a problem like that, you can't completely relax. But I realized that I could make choices. I could choose to despair or I could choose, to the best of my ability, to keep my mind fixed on the joy of each day as I lived it. I recalled the words of Isaiah 26:3. "Thou wilt keep him in perfect peace, whose mind is stayed on thee: because he trusteth in thee." And I prayed to God to strengthen my resolve to trust in Him, no matter what.

At the end of August I returned to Dr. Rossman. Neither of us mentioned Dr. Karik. I spoke to Dr. Rossman about a red spot on my palate and general irritation of the palate. He looked at it and said, "It can't be irritation from the surgery. Don't worry about it. You're closed up now. Go back to school." He advised me to return every six months for a checkup.

Again I asked him about the biopsy on the tenth of July.

"I never did a biopsy," he said. "There was no biopsy."

"How can you say that to me?" I said. "How can you deny it?"

"It's my word against yours," he replied.

I never saw Dr. Rossman professionally again.

The next day I returned to Lehigh for the fall semester and my final year in attendance there. In addition to math, science, and history courses, I took an elective in psychology.

It concerned me that I tired so easily. I hoped that some of this was due to anxiety. As any cancer patient knows, it isn't easy to live in the shadow of six-month checkups. They tie you down to the disease, and you must find some way to keep on going without letting this dominate your living. Dr. Karik had told me everything appeared to be fine, but he admonished me to contact him immediately if I noticed any change in my mouth

or in the little red spot that had been on my palate even before
I had left Dr. Rossman's care. It was difficult not to dwell on my
illness and at the same time be constantly aware of it so that I
could monitor that spot. I felt as if I were walking a kind of
tightrope: the slightest change and over I could go—to cancer.

That Christmas vacation I went to Yale–New Haven Memorial Hospital for a CAT scan. Dr. Karik was now practicing and
teaching there. Once again I was told that everything appeared
to be fine. By this time, other than for some irritation in the
upper portion of my mouth that never seemed to improve, and
the little red spot that remained constant, my mouth had
healed. I could eat and drink normally. And I no longer had
pain. My energy level improved tremendously, and I was confident that I had nothing to worry about so far as the cancer was
concerned. I thought I had it licked.

One day in early February, Sally Lathers, one of the girls in
my dorm apartment, told me that she was putting on a fashion
show to raise money for the J. F. Goodwin Scholarship Fund.
"Invite your parents," she said. "Tell your friends. We need
the money."

Sally was a pretty girl from the West Indies, and I liked her
a lot.

"I'll do more than come," I said. "I'd like to be in it."

She raised her eyebrows and stared at me. "Do you know
what the J. F. Goodwin Scholarship Fund is?" she asked.

"No!" I replied truthfully. "I never heard of it."

"I thought so." Her dark eyes grew intense. "It's for schol-
arships and grants for *black* students."

When I said nothing, she continued.

"It's sponsored by the *black* student union of Lehigh."

"So?" I shrugged. "Can I be in it?"

" Yeah." She grinned. "But you're going to be the only white
person in it."

On March 2, my parents drove over to see the show. "I'm so
glad we came, Bea," Dad said. "It was wonderful!" He looked

at the program. " 'A Touch of Class,' " he read. "It really was. You looked beautiful!"

The show had been a success, and I was so happy for all of the people who had worked so hard, every day, for more than a month. It had been my first extracurricular activity since my previous surgery. My happiness was more than for the fashion show. It was also for me, for my freedom from cancer.

Sometime that spring, Ann Marie Shoeman, M.D., senior associate dean of Medical College of Pennsylvania, interviewed me to reappraise my acceptance into the medical college. We had an instant rapport. "I see no reason why you shouldn't continue in the program," she told me at the end of the interview. That day, she was one of the most important persons in my life, and somehow I believe that she empathized with me enough to know that. All through medical school she continued to be a staunch friend, and she will always hold a very special place in my heart. She never lost faith in me, and her thoughtfulness helped me over some very rough times.

Before leaving Lehigh, each student in the six-year program had the opportunity to stay overnight with a medical student at MCP and to attend the medical college with that student on the following day. In this way, we got a firsthand taste of what the future held for us. Immediately upon my arrival at my medical student's apartment, I was impressed with the volume of books and medical journals. Up at 5 A.M., we didn't get back to her apartment until 8 P.M. She was on the go hour after hour, making rounds, listening to morning reports, caring for patients, drawing bloods. As I watched her at work, I said to myself, "Oh, I'll never be able to do all this. How can anybody keep up this pace?" That night, when I got back to Lehigh, I felt so tired that I thought I was going to die. Now, years later, I'm glad that I didn't know that there was such a thing as "call," where interns and residents work around the clock and into the following day at a hectic pace—a thirty-six-hour steady work shift, sometimes with one or two hours of sleep, sometimes with none. Those who were wiser than we knew that we had to be broken into the real state of the art gradually. You just can't jump into it. You go through a preparation period.

After that, the weeks continued to fly by, but not fast enough for me. I loved Lehigh, but I could hardly wait to begin my studies at MCP.

My preclinical adviser, Dr. Cynthia Hart, asked me what my goals were in medical school. I told her that I was interested in nerve regeneration, and she suggested that I contact Dr. Charles Goldstein, the chairman of anatomy at MCP.

When I went to see Dr. Goldstein at his office, there was a chemistry between us and I liked him instantly. I sensed immediately that he was a very kind man. Middle-aged, with dark hair and bright, piercing eyes. His office door was open and he stood up from his desk to greet me. "Beatrice Engstrand?"

"Yes."

"Come in. Come in." He held out his hand in greeting and then indicated a chair near him. "Sit down." He came directly to the point. "What makes you think you'd be interested in nerve regeneration research?"

I had often thought about that question, so my answer was ready. "It has always bothered me to know that nerve cells can't grow back if they are damaged." I remembered my conversations with Dr. Glickmann, dean emeritus of the College of Physicians and Surgeons at Columbia University, who had befriended me and often chatted informally with me about the field of medicine. "When I talked about this with Dr. Glickmann, he told me that if someone had a simple spinal cord injury, if his spinal cord was cut, he couldn't move. Shortly before his death, when I was about to enter my six-year medical program, Dr. Glickmann encouraged me to consider the field of neurology. It troubled me that even with a simple lesion, a simple abnormality like that, a person couldn't walk. I said that there must be an answer somewhere as to how to make these cells grow back."

"Do you know anything about research?"

"No, I don't."

"Let me tell you," he said soberly. "Research is a long and arduous process. It takes many years, even many lifetimes, to get results. The pacemaker concept was first devised way back in the seventeen hundreds. Do you realize that this is the first generation ever to use it? And do you realize that these ideas we have now may not be used until two hundred years in the future?" He paused to let that sink in, then continued. "Research is not immediate gratification. A researcher picks and gnaws at little things, gradually hoping to contribute. And if he's lucky, he will see results in his lifetime. If it's like the Salk vaccine, he would be around when the time comes for that one research item to come to fruition."

By the time the interview ended, we agreed that I would work with him that summer, learning basic research techniques. Summers thereafter I would continue to do more research with him until I finally progressed to the point where I could contribute significantly to the project. That was my original aim in medical school.

My time at Lehigh was drawing to an end. Chit was going to fly to Thailand for his vacation. But first he spent a week at my parents' home. On the day of his flight, I drove him to Kennedy Airport. He had become increasingly concerned about my move to MCP.

"You'll forget me, Bea."

"No, I won't."

"Yes, you will. You'll get involved with all those doctors and medical students over there and you'll grow away from me."

"I won't."

"Then tell me now that you'll become engaged to me. I want to know that you won't date anyone else."

"I can't do that," I said. "I must complete medical school before I can do anything like that. I don't know what the world holds in store for me, where I'll be guided to go, what I'll be guided to do—what new people I may meet. You don't know either. You don't have your Ph.D. yet. You have no idea where you will be working or what kind of a job you will get. We are too unsettled to tie ourselves down yet."

"I'm going to lose you, Bea," he said sadly. "I know it."

At Kennedy Airport, I watched while his plane took off. And I continued to watch until it became a faint speck in the distance and disappeared into the clouds.

My studies at Lehigh ended on May 17, 1980. After a brief vacation at home, I looked forward to moving into my Philadelphia apartment and to commencing my medical training.

# Chapter Seven

In June 1980 I moved to my apartment in Philadelphia. I started research and looked forward to my studies at the Medical College of Pennsylvania.

Every morning I drove to the basic science building in the main hospital at MCP and reported to Dr. Goldstein's technician. Polly always greeted me with a cheerful smile, and I appreciated her willingness to instruct me. In the beginning, she gave me an overview of the lab work. After that, much of my time during the day was spent working at the computer and counting cells and neurons under the microscope, doing research on neurotransmitters and nervous system development.

Unknown to me then, my life was to be interrupted by the death of my grandmother and by another bout with cancer. But now I was preparing for a return trip to Long Island to visit my grandmother. Mom had just phoned to say that Grandma was ill.

The last afternoon sun poured through the opened slats of the venetian blinds and streamed into my kitchen and living room. I got up from the kitchen table and adjusted them so that I could still look out but without the glare. Then I kicked off my shoes, poured myself a mug of hot coffee, and sat down again.

The kitchen and living room looked out onto the courtyard with its scattering of fruit trees in rich green leaf. I sighed, contented. Like any new neighborhood, this would take some getting used to at first. But I knew that I was going to like living here for the four years that I would be studying at MCP. My bedroom windows looked out onto the largest black oak tree I had ever seen and, beyond that, into the grounds of the Germantown Cricket Club.

I'd lived here less than two months, and already I felt settled. It was that kind of community. There was a nice mix of people in the apartment complex—a wide variety of ethnic groups. Some were newcomers as I was. Others were families that had lived here for a quarter-century and more. And in the fall, when the school year started, there would be medical students, too.

It all seemed so peaceful, but as with any big city, I thought, you had to use caution and be alert, especially if you had to be out alone after dark. That was why my parents had gone to a kennel and bought Sabrina for me. I looked down at her now, sleeping. Her square muzzle rested against my feet. A full-grown rottweiler, gentle, dependable, fiercely protective. She'd taken to me instantly. The first night I'd moved into the apartment, Mom and Dad had driven over in two cars. Mom and I arrived first, and as we entered the apartment building, in the few seconds that it took us to find the unfamiliar light switch, a man sneaked behind us through the open door and into the basement. Only my screams saved us from personal attack. Neighbors rushed out thinking there was a fire, and the man escaped. Dad and Mom bought Sabrina for me after that. She was thoroughly trained and obedient, but she was death on cats. So my cats Lehigh and Whiskers returned home to live with my parents.

Sabrina lay in the back-seat during the drive home. At times my eyes clouded with tears. I brushed them away with the back of my hand and continued the long drive toward home.

Grandma, Mom's mother, was dying. One part of me knew this and accepted it. Another part of me found Grandma's approaching death totally unbelievable. She had always been the very personification of life.

Many times in her early seventies, Grandma had said, "Beatrice, I'm going to live to be a hundred and we'll have a big party." We had had a lot of fun talking about what a very big party that would be. She liked big parties and so did I. She had tremendous vitality, a life that encompassed both positive and negative in extremes but never in an even balance, never canceling itself out. It was hard to believe that now I was driving home to see her for the very last time.

*Grandma had had everything*, I thought. *And she had thrown it all up in the air.*

She had been a world-renowned beauty in the early 1920s. But she had never sought fame. Fame had sought her. Her face had been so strikingly beautiful that noted artists who saw her walking about Manhattan rushed to present their cards to her. Herbert Adams had done a marble bust and paintings of her in 1924, and Quinn, sculptures in gold and in marble. She had been starred in silent educational films for the Fox Film Studios.

Emil Fuchs, friend and favorite artist of the British royal family, had been completely captivated by my grandmother's beauty. One of many distinguished admirers, he had proposed marriage to her and she had rejected him. But she remained his favorite model. And it was her face and her neck and her shoulders that he had sculpted into the pink marble bust of *A Modern Juno* that he had exhibited at the Fine Arts Galleries and at the National Academy of Design. *A Modern Juno* had made its debut in the museum of the Hispanic Society in 1923 for the national exhibition of American sculpture. More than five hundred works of art had been represented there under the auspices of Archer Huntington, distinguished art collector.

According to *The Evening Telegram*, March 26, 1923, which

carried a photograph of *A Modern Juno*, art critics, gathered for a preview in Mr. Fuchs's studio at the Beaux Arts Building, declared, "She will be the sensation of the hour. Nothing has been done like her either in line or in feeling. So closely does she follow the trend of the ancient Greek that it is difficult to believe she is modelled from life, that her counterpart lives and breathes and moves right here. . . ."

I had read Grandma's clippings over and over and over again, so many times that I knew most of them by heart. Grandma herself had never paid much attention to them. When I was a young child, I had come across them in an old cardboard box hidden away in her attic.

"Grandma, what's this?" I had asked, indicating the opened box packed with pictures and papers.

"Oh, that!" She dismissed the contents with a shrug. "Nothing very interesting. Just some old pictures of me that Great-Grandma kept." Mom, seeing that they were in danger of being destroyed, asked Grandma if she could have them. "Of course," Grandma said, not much concerned. She had turned to me. "Would you like to play dolls, Beatrice?"

Grandma made an ideal playmate. She always saw things from a child's perspective. She was brilliant and gifted but she had a simplicity about her, a Peter Pan quality. She could make up stories and play dolls better than any little friend I had, thread a worm when fishing with Don, or shoot an arrow straight to the target.

It was two months since she had phoned me in Philadelphia on her seventy-eighth birthday. "I'm in the hospital." Then, as if to soften the blow, she had added cheerfully, "Don't worry. It's nothing. My gallbladder, that's all."

"Oh, Grandma," I had said, horrified. "I hope you don't die."

And she had replied, "Oh, I hope I do! What a way to go! Under anesthesia, you get put out of your misery and that's it."

But she had lived through the surgery and the results were totally unexpected. The surgeon had opened her up and closed her again without removing anything. She had primary cancer of the gallbladder, which had metastasized to the liver and to the pancreas. For the first two weeks after surgery, Grandma made statements that belied her illness, and it was obvious that she didn't want us to correct her. We respected her wishes, taking our cues from her questions. When she asked a question, we answered truthfully. But when she chose the option of chemotherapy, she whispered, "If I go for the treatments, I may be able to live through the summer." After that she didn't discuss the prognosis. She wouldn't allow the disease to monopolize the last two months of her life. Instead, she encouraged her friends and family to talk about themselves. She wanted to know about the things we were doing and about our plans for the future.

I had been with Grandma when Mom drove her to the hospital for her last chemotherapy treatment. In the car, heaves continually wracked her body. Mom intuitively changed course and stopped at Crab Meadow Beach. She pulled the car up close to the picnic stand, then to the boardwalk—just for a moment. Grandma lifted her head slightly and turned her face toward the large rocks bordering the inlet, toward the wooden pagoda ending the boardwalk, toward the whitecaps breaking near shore. It had been here that she had met my grandfather and had finally lost her heart.

My grandfather had been a cold, hard man. I had met him only once, before I was grown. There had been a wildness in him that even a beauty such as hers couldn't tame. But still she had loved him, and remembering that love comforted her now.

She reached into her purse and took out a small sepia photograph taken on their honeymoon. They looked young and happy, seated in a carriage drawn by a palomino wearing a funny little straw hat decked with flowers. Grandma held it up for me to see and then carefully replaced it in her purse.

"It's a beautiful picture, Grandma," I said.

She smiled, pleased.

This was the picture that she chose to carry about with her

because of him. But I remembered other pictures of her that I had seen on magazine covers: *Redbook, Theatre, Motor Boating, Hearst's International.* There had been many others, she said when I had questioned her. But she hadn't bothered to keep them.

When we reached the hospital, Grandma invited me into the chemotherapy room. "You're going to study medicine, Bea," she said. "You might as well see what this is all about."

I asked her doctor how the chemotherapy was going to be used.

"For palliative treatment only," he said quietly.

*Palliative!* I thought. *She's vomiting her head off. Is this really going to help her?*

They gave her a little and then stopped. She wasn't able to go through it.

They admitted her that day and advised us to leave because they would be working with her. A few days after that she was able to leave the hospital. But she had had to go right back, sooner even than her doctor had expected. I telephoned every day from Philadelphia, but Grandma kept putting my visits off. She didn't want me to see her looking so ill. Whenever Dad visited her, she would confide in him that she was concerned about me. She didn't believe that all of my cancer had been gotten out. And then, one day when I telephoned, she said that she would look forward to seeing me on my next day off. And I knew instinctively that this would be the last time I would ever see her. "I'll be there this weekend," I had said.

And now, this was that weekend.

Grandma was an adventurer. She took gambles. These didn't always work out, but at least she was true to herself. "Be true to yourself, Beatrice," she had said. "Don't be stilted. Life is meant to be lived, to be enjoyed." She let me know that there are those who don't enjoy life because they allow themselves to become too entrapped with the complexities of living.

Her faith was very simple. She trusted in God to meet her

every need. And she was always happiest when she could be of help to others.

But, she wasn't all sweetness and light. She was a woman of contrasts. She enjoyed a fight and liked to create unrest, excitement. She was both elegant and simple, rich and poor all in one woman. She gave me a taste of the Bohemian and a special spirit of living.

When I walked down the long hospital corridor to Grandma's room at the very end of the hall, it was nearly ten o'clock in the morning. I would be the only person to visit her that day. That was the way Grandma wanted it.

I found her sitting in a chair, waiting for me. Her snow-white hair had been freshly arranged and her beautiful face held an expression of tranquility.

We spent most of the day shoring up memories against the ravages of time. I asked her about our family background and wrote her answers down. Her mother's family had been Lutheran, Methodist, and Quaker. Ministers, attorneys, and statesmen, they had been surprisingly less rigid than her father's family, who had all been physicians with the exception of her father, who had been a dental surgeon. He was graduated from the University of Pennsylvania Dental College and had been a fellow of the C. N. Pierce Dental Society. Her uncle had been an ophthalmologist; her grandfather, a general practitioner; her great uncle, an obstetrician. Their forebears in Stuttgart, Germany, went back to Baron von Kummerle. In America, they had changed their family name to Kamerly.

She spoke of their dedication, telling me how, at times, they would get paid in eggs or chickens or not at all. And how they always kept current with the latest developments in their fields.

I spoke then of Poppy's father and of his devotion to his patients.

"When the peasants had no money to pay for care," I said, "they embroidered tablecloths and other linens for him. And when he died, all of the newspapers were bordered in black.

The King of Sweden sent emissaries to purchase the linens for the royal family because they were national heirlooms."

I smiled at her. "Your father and the doctors in your family and Poppy's father were storybook heroes to me."

"Once I thought of becoming a surgeon," Grandma said. "But I didn't stick with it. You did."

She expressed interest in my work at the lab. I explained the purpose of the research and my very small part in it. "I may not continue working in research," I said. "I think my gift of healing lies in clinical work, caring directly for the patients."

In spite of the sad occasion, we spent a glorious day together. And such was the strength of her spirit that I almost forgot at times why I was there.

Her face glowed with pride as she introduced me to each shift of nurses. "This is my granddaughter. She's in Philadelphia studying to be a doctor."

The nurses would smile at her, their eyes filled with compassion. "That's wonderful," they said.

The last shift looked across the room at me and smiled politely. I knew that they were waiting for me to leave so they could settle her for the night. But Grandma asked them to let us have just a few more minutes alone.

We each studied the other's face intently. Then I reached over and stroked my fingers through her baby-fine white hair.

Grandma's voice was whisper soft. "Bea! I'm very proud of you. And I want you to keep going with your work. Don't come back to see me again if anything should happen."

There were a few days of orientation at MCP before medical classes formally began. This was the first opportunity that any of us had had to meet our fellow classmates in one group that hereafter would be known as the Class of 1984. There were about 110 students, two Ph.D.s, a wide variety of ages. The youngest in the class came from the six-year program and were about twenty years old; the oldest student in the class was about the age of forty-one.

Genetics, anatomy, statistics, psychiatry, nutrition! This is the stuff of which dreams are made, I thought, when I learned what our first courses would be.

The first weeks of classes I received honors on the first round of exams, liked all of the professors, and thought that my classmates were great.

"Wow! God," I said silently, talking to Him directly, "I'm really here!"

Chit returned from Thailand and visited me as often as he could. We were having problems with our relationship because he feared that I was growing away from him and that I thought more of my new friends than I did of him. And worry about my health hung over both of us like a damp cloud. The little red spot in my mouth wasn't gone, and I wasn't feeling well. And I was concerned about Grandma. I didn't want to burden my parents, especially Mom. She visited Grandma every day, and I knew that Grandma was failing rapidly now. But Chit insisted that I tell them about my mouth.

"Don't be a fool, Bea," he said. "Cancer is serious." And so I phoned Mom.

Dr. Karik scheduled me for a biopsy in his office at Yale–New Haven Memorial Hospital, early in that coming September.

Grandma died about a month after my visit to her. She had wasted away and fallen into a coma, but she had died with dignity. No extraordinary measures had been taken. I didn't attend her funeral. Mom said that Grandma had mentioned several times that she didn't want me to miss school other than to take care of my health. And so I stayed in Philadelphia and sat for a test on the day of Grandma's funeral. It wasn't an easy thing to do, but she had wanted it that way, and it was my memorial to her.

The day after Grandma's funeral, Mom drove me to Yale–New Haven for my biopsy. Dr. Karik numbed my mouth and removed a little bit of tissue. It wasn't a painful procedure this time, and I didn't even need stitches. *This is such a simple procedure*, I thought. *How important can this be?* But it bothered me that Dr. Karik didn't give me a look of reassurance. He appeared to be as friendly as ever, but there was something serious about his demeanor that puzzled me.

As we drove back to Philadelphia, Mom announced that she would stay with me until the biopsy report came in. She said that the change of scenery would be restful for her. Now, knowing the tremendous pressure she was under, I don't know how she managed to keep a cheerful face most of the time. And whenever I would catch her looking sad, she would say that she had been thinking of Grandma.

Exactly one week after Grandma's death, one week after my biopsy, and one week before my surgery, when I did not as yet know the biopsy results, I had a very vivid dream. In this dream, I walked into my kitchen in Philadelphia and sat down, face to face with Grandma. It was nighttime. Mom was sleeping in her bedroom. Grandma looked at me and I got chills.

I said, "You're dead."

And Grandma said with a very firm voice, which was unusual for her, "I'm here to talk to you. You will be going through a period when you will be experiencing severe pain. Pain, Beatrice, pain," she emphasized.

I panicked. I said, "Grandma, I can't."

And she said, "You have to. I did it. I went through severe, agonizing pain and I got through it, and so will you."

"But you died," I said. And she sort of smiled at me. I asked her if she was in pain now. She stared at me and didn't answer. That was a pretty big message for a person who just died to give. I woke up convinced that I had met with her, and I was startled by her message. I didn't know what pain she was talking about, but I knew that Grandma was telling me that some terrible ordeal lay ahead of me and that I could get through it if I only had the determination to keep on going.

That week Mom's father also appeared to me in a dream. He told me that he was sorry that I would have to suffer so much and that I would not be seeing him anymore. Then he asked me to forgive him for the mean things he had done. I forgave him and he immediately disappeared. I awoke from that dream happy that he had found peace.

The third person to visit me in a psychic dream that week was Dad's mom. She had died of cancer shortly before Dad's seventeenth birthday. In the dream, she introduced herself to me. "I'm your father's mother," she said. "And I just came to tell you that I care. You won't be seeing me again."

And then on Friday, October 3, I received the biopsy results. Mucoepidermoid cancer! Immediate surgery required! Mutilation!

# Chapter Eight

It was Monday night, October 6, 1980. I was bracing myself for the surgery at Yale–New Haven Memorial Hospital. My parents were with me in my room when I had a stream of visitors. The first was a young male intern who came in and sat by my bed. As we chatted, I could tell that he found me attractive. I wondered if anyone would ever again think of me as attractive after that night.

Then Dr. Karik's assistant came and described the surgery to me. He said he hoped they would not have to remove my left eye, but it was a definite possibility. I was stunned. No mention had been made of this surgical procedure. I demanded an explanation from Dr. Karik when he came in to say good night. He assured me that he would do everything possible to spare my eye, but he could not know for sure until the operation was under way. He would have to remove my left upper jaw, gum, teeth, cheekbone, and palate. Before taking the sleeping pills from the nurse, I looked into a mirror and said good-bye to myself as I had known me. I had just turned twenty years old.

That night, waiting for sleep to come, I felt utterly helpless. Before in my life if I wanted to change something about myself—lose weight, change clothing style—I could do it. But now my body faced a battle to overcome an illness that threatened life itself. And I lived in that body, it and I inseparable. My mind, intact, remained chained to this body afflicted with this dread illness. Therefore, I, too, must face this battle. With God's help, I determined to fight. But it wasn't going to be easy.

Every waking moment felt overshadowed by this peril. And many things assumed new meaning. I recalled my high school graduation and how I had finally become valedictorian. No longer to me now were grades of B unsatisfactory. I realized that whatever I achieved in a particular day, whatever my daily activities might be, represented the best I could do at that moment in time. I thought of Beth and of her tragic death. I longed for a second chance to appreciate life more—to give to it something that showed my appreciation.

In the morning, as I awoke from sleep wishing to escape from the torment of my dreams, I realized that the real nightmare I faced was reality itself. Dr. Karik had advised my parents to visit me that morning, and they arrived just in time to kiss me good-bye as I was being wheeled to the operating room. I knew they would be praying for me, and I trusted God to hear their prayers.

After surgery, when I woke up from the operation, I felt paralyzed. I didn't know that I was in a cast. I couldn't see and I couldn't speak. I felt trapped in this dark void. I felt scared, lonely, afraid that I was going to die. I could hear an alarm bell go off every time I kept going in and out of panic episodes.

The intensive care nurse came to me and said, "Your head is in a cast. It is like a cast you have on a leg. Don't worry, we know you can't talk. We know you can't move." That helped me to realize that somebody knew how I was doing.

When my parents first saw me in the intensive care unit, my

entire head was in a cast, except for the mouth. Both eyes were covered with bandages, my mouth was full of gauze, and mucous streams clogged my throat. Much of the surgery had been performed from the inside after the doctors sliced open my face, stretching the flaps of skin, cutting out the bones, nerves, muscles, and connective tissues, then stitching together the thin outer flaps of the cheek to make a covering over the hollow. I was attached to a multiplicity of machines. A skin graft had been taken from one buttock to restructure the contours of my face.

Mom said, "Try to move your finger if you can respond at all." So I concentrated on my finger and was able to move it. Mom and I were able to establish a little communication that way.

After several days, I was placed in a private room. The head cast was still on, but the resident came in and removed half of it, leaving one side of my head in a cast and the other side not. My left eye was sewn shut with black thread. A tube was inserted through my nose down to my stomach for liquid feedings. This, too, was painful because my nose had been cut up. I could barely distinguish light from dark, and we didn't know how much sight would come back to my "good" eye.

Gradually, over a period of days, shapeless, shadowy forms emerged. But my sense of smell was gone and my hearing impaired. The entire left side of my face was grotesquely swollen. The artificially rounded contours and the bunching of my cheek where it had been re-joined to my face, the droop of my mouth, the drooling—all gave me the appearance of a retarded child.

The nurses were not familiar with the special care I required, so they had to be personally instructed by Dr. Karik. Day after day, my mother sat at my bedside from early morning until almost midnight, suctioning mucous every few minutes from my mouth and throat. Every couple of days there would be a milestone of sorts, when some of the gauze bandaging my head and face would be removed or changed. Physicians from other floors and other departments in the hospital came to look at me, curious about the technique that had been used.

I refused most pain medication after the surgery even though the pain was almost unbearable. I did not want to cloud my brain. I insisted upon studying. My medical textbooks were near my bedside, and Mom read them to me. MCP professors compiled homework and notes. True to his word, Dr. Fein forwarded them to me at the hospital. It was a futile attempt at learning, because I would doze in and out of consciousness, waken to gag on mucous, and experience pain so great that I could not remember what had been read to me. Still, I insisted that the reading continue. My dream of becoming a doctor and of graduating on time with my class inspired me to fight on.

The love of friends also provided much strength. One day as my mother read to me, flowers arrived, a gift from my medical school classmates. "Beatrice, they're long-stemmed roses. Yellow, your favorite color." I could not see them or smell them, but I reached out my hand to feel the soft petals.

Chit visited, bringing a large, colorful poster of a brown puppy that Maria had circulated about the Lehigh campus. The poster was packed full of notes and get-well wishes. And MCP classmates and professors kept up a steady stream of cards and letters. All of these were Scotch-taped to the walls of my room until we ran out of wall space. Then they were laid in a neat pile on my night table.

Now, in looking back and trying to assess the things that helped me cope, I think that it was important that none of the cards was read just once and then taped to the walls in order to decorate the room. Each card was put to work many times. On days that my mail was lighter than usual, Mom reread some of them. She always found something new to say about the picture on the card or the thought conveyed in the message. And she talked to me about the person who had sent the card. It didn't matter that she had never met the person. She would tell me who had sent the card and then say something such as, "This is such a pretty card, filled with pictures of little frogs sitting on a lily pad. John must have spent a great deal of time looking for something very special for you . . . What lovely handwriting Debbie has . . . Here's someone who really misses you. Listen to the letter he wrote."

I think that those constant messages and that continuous outpouring of love served as a kind of umbilical cord, a kind of lifeline keeping me attached to the real world. They helped me to hold on to my identity. And their good effect was compounded as Mom read each of them to me over and over again. This kept me constantly aware that my identity was intact, that my friends and peers still recognized me as myself and would welcome me back.

During all of this time I still saw only light and shadows with my good eye. And then one morning I sensed unusual excitement in my room. Dr. Karik and a resident removed the stitches from my left eye. I cried when they were removed, because I couldn't see at all and I was sure I was blind. But then after a few minutes I responded to the light of a flashlight, and we knew that my vision would gradually return. But we didn't know to what extent.

After the first week I was able to get out of bed and walk around the hospital halls, leaning on my mother for support. Progress was slow, but we kept at it. When I was able to walk the distance of two corridors, Mom was elated. It reminded me of the time when I had been a child and she had encouraged me to walk the distance of a telephone pole.

My parents and I had been told that we would probably have to wait another week to ten days for the pathology report. That evening a slender, attractive man in his late twenties or early thirties rapped at my door. His face was wreathed in smiles. "May I come in?" he asked. "I'm an evangelical pastor."

"Of course," Dad said. "Please come in."

Still smiling, he walked over to my bed and offered his hand to me. Then he shook hands with Dad and Mom. I was relieved that he didn't stare at me in horrified fascination as so many people had, even other patients. "One of my parishioners is a patient here," he explained. He turned to me. "She saw you groping through the halls with your mother and asked if I would visit you. Since you are far from home, I might be of some comfort." We told him that we were waiting for the pathology report but that it wouldn't be ready for at least another week.

"Oh, yes, it will be!" he said positively. "You will hear tomorrow morning and it will be good!" He turned to me. "Sister, you have nothing to fear. Trust in the Lord." We all joined hands and prayed together. Then he read passages from the Bible. "Pray, sister," he said to me as he was leaving. "Pray all night long without stopping and with faith."

"I can't do that," I protested. "I'm a sick person and I need my sleep."

"God's energy will keep you going," he said. "And then tomorrow you will hear good things. Only believe!"

After that, Dad drove back to Long Island, and Mom returned to her motel room. I was all alone with the fear of death. The phone rang, and the welcome voice of a fellow six-year student broke the silent stillness. I asked him if he thought I was going to die. He said he didn't know but he was praying for me.

Alone, in the quiet darkness of my room, I realized that I was close to death. I lay on my bed with my eyes open and prayed all night. I prayed the Lord's Prayer and the Twenty-third Psalm and other prayers. And again, I had the feeling that there were many dead people in the room with me in spirit. I prayed all that night. And I finally received an inner peace when I realized that I had done all that I could do. And then I let go and I let God! The next day, Dr. Karik received the pathology report—the cancer was gone.

I no longer feared death, but there was another horror to

contend with. The gauze packing that temporarily filled in the gaping hole where the roof of my mouth had previously been would have to be removed. One side of my face was hollow, and I feared that my face would cave in. The packing, saturated with blood and pus, helped to stem the bleeding and to support the surrounding tissues. With the gauze in place, I was able to speak and also to deny the extent of my deformity. Although this was not the purpose of the packing, I had discovered that it could serve as a crude sounding board. Little by little, working with the packing in place, my speech became intelligible. But one afternoon not long after that, my surgeon told me that the packing was to be removed the next day. He warned me that with the packing removed, I would no longer have any sounding board and that speech would be impossible.

I had not been told that I would never again be able to speak intelligibly unless I was wearing a specially designed, custom-made prosthesis. And at this early period of recovery from surgery, I had no prosthesis.

After the packing was removed, physicians from other floors and other departments came to look at me, curious about the results of this unique surgery. Big mucous secretions continued to fall down from the surgery site. I needed to be suctioned with a long, rubberlike tube that Mom or the nurses had to use every few minutes because I couldn't breathe. They had to be extremely careful that the suction didn't pull the grafting on the inside of my cheek.

And now a new horror began. I tried to speak but could not. Only sounds of air and unintelligible raspings escaped from me. My mouth felt as though it had been blown away with a short-barreled shotgun.

I panicked. My movements restricted by tubes and skin grafting, one of my arms strapped to a board which held it steady for an IV, my hands clenched and unclenched.

But through it all, Mom stayed beside me. "It's going to be all right, Bea. It's going to be all right," she repeated over and over again. "We'll get a good prosthesis for you and then you'll be able to talk again." I felt the soft touch of her fingertips stroking my restricted arm. Continuing to talk to me, she walked to my other side, and taking my free hand in her own, she brought it up to her lips and kissed it. She placed a pencil in my hand. "Write, Bea," she said. She positioned my hand on a notebook. From then on, I communicated either by writing short sentences or by making gestures.

And then I remembered the technique I had used to ventriloquize with "Uncle Bunny." I determined to try it. At first, the sounds coming from me were ten times more garbled than those of the impaired children for whom I had performed. I remembered how I had struggled to understand them in order that they might communicate with me. Now I knew that if I just kept on trying, Mom would keep on struggling to understand me. She would never tire of trying to help me find a way out of my horrible entrapment.

Finally, after hours of frustration, despair, and exhaustive effort, I tried my skill on Dr. Karik during his morning rounds. As he turned to leave, I ventriloquized a word. It was muffled and without volume, but it was a word. Startled, he turned back to me.

"How did you do that?" he asked. He came closer to me.

I pointed to my throat.

"Do it again," he said.

I repeated it.

"I forgot that you are a ventriloquist," he said. "Good for you. It's not very clear, but it's something."

Mirrors were kept away from my room. Each day Mom assured me that I was looking better. It must have been very difficult for her to keep my spirits bolstered and yet not overdo it, so that I would not have too great a letdown when I first saw myself.

From the initial shock, my mother gently guided me back to laughter by reassuring me that my appearance was improving constantly. She read Norman Cousins's *Anatomy of an Illness*, the Bible, and other inspirational writing to keep up her own spirits so that she could be cheerful for me when I was awake.

Mom feared that each year, October 7, the day of my surgery, would be a day of horrible memories for me. And so, looking to the future, she and Dad impressed upon me that October 7 was a special kind of birthday for me. They gave me a birthday card, dating it 10/7/80. The card read, "I'm tickled pink it's your birthday!" Dad wrote: "Dear Bea, Oct. 7th is your second birthday—the day you start your new life with complete health. You are truly a wonderful person who is going to be a great person. Dad loves you very, very much and will always love and be very proud of you. Love, Dad XXXX." And Mom wrote: "Dear Doctor Beatrice Engstrand, I am so very happy and so very grateful to be able to share this momentous day with you—the beginning of a completely healthy life filled with all the many joys which you so richly deserve. Now! *Move forward* continuously toward your cherished career! Love forever, Mommy XXX."

One day Aunt Addie drove with Dad all the way from the United Presbyterian Residence on Long Island to my hospital room. She talked to me and expressed her love. Then we held hands and both of us fell asleep—I, on my bed, and she, sitting in the stuffed leather chair beside my bed with her head resting on a pillow. It did me good to see this beloved old person, because I knew how very much her friendship had contributed to my life, and I appreciated the effort that she had made to be of help to me now. Her effort inspired me. And it helped me to believe that I could still contribute, too.

Every morning and every afternoon Dr. Karik visited me. In his chats with me, he'd talk about my career and about things that I should do and shouldn't do when I became a physician. He continued to accept me as a physician-in-training, which helped me to keep my dream alive. And his positive attitude helped me to retain my identity. He dressed impeccably, almost daily wearing a different sport jacket. When I complimented him about this, he told me that it is important for a physician to dress well and that I should remember that when I had my practice. At first he tried to encourage me to take a year off from my medical studies in order to recuperate. But when he saw how much they meant to me, he accepted my decision to return to school, and encouraged me.

Reentering the "real world" was traumatic. Dr. Karik released me from the hospital shortly after the surgery to see a prosthodontist. On the way, the taxi driver expressed sympathy, saying, "Oh, I'm sorry you were hit by a Mack truck."

The prosthodontist did not know what, if anything, he could do for me. "It would have been much easier to make a prosthesis if your eye had been removed," he said. "Then we would have had something on which to hook the prosthesis." In a state of near hysteria, I returned to the hospital.

Another day, Dr. Karik suggested that buying a new outfit would pick up my spirits. People in the nearby department store openly stared at me. Some laughed. I felt like the Hunchback of Notre Dame because I couldn't speak. My mother found a sales clerk and enlisted her sympathy by explaining that I had just come from the hospital and must go right back. The clerk brought me a chair, because I was too weak to stand very long. Because I am very tall and slender, most off-the-rack clothes do not fit me correctly. However, fit was not important then; my vision was too poor to tell the difference. Mom, eager to do anything to help, reasoned that if one dress would lift my spirits, seven dresses would send them aloft. Over the next several days, when I was up to it, she dressed me in the new clothes. The nurses were very supportive, stopping by to see the dresses and complimenting me on the way I looked. This did a great deal to give me the courage to face the outside world and to prepare for my return to medical school.

But before I could return to school, I needed an artificial jaw in order to speak intelligibly, to eat, to drink. It was difficult to find a prosthodontist capable of doing this work because I had no bone left on which to hook the prosthesis. I made several tiring trips to Manhattan. (Too weak to sit up in the car, I lay in the backseat propped up with pillows.) I hoped that a prosthodontist would put me back together again—that a prosthesis would return me to normal.

On my first trip to the prosthodontist, he couldn't put an impression in. My mouth wouldn't open the width of one finger. He gave me a pyramid-shaped crowbar with grooves. I was to insert this into my mouth, twist it, and try to crank my mouth open for six hours a day for many months that year. I had to get to use my mouth and face muscles again so that I could open my mouth wide enough to be worked on. I got the device that day and practiced with it from then on.

The following week, the prosthodonist was able to take impressions. After that, he filed down all my top teeth on the right side of my mouth and all the bottom teeth in one sitting and put temporary crowns on. There were no teeth or gums on the upper left side. These procedures were very painful because the tissues and nerve endings of my mouth had been so traumatized. But it was worthwhile, because he constructed a temporary prosthesis. This helped to seal up the hole and gave me a tooth in the front so I looked a little more acceptable. The prosthesis rocked and felt very unsteady, but it allowed me to eat soft foods, such as yogurt, ice cream, custard, and Jell-O, into which Mom mixed several natural vitamins, minerals, and protein supplements. And it also served as a model for a permanent prosthesis made later by Dr. Bal Singh of the University of Pennsylvania.

The prosthesis I now wear looks somewhat like a denture, but with gum tissue, and is contoured to fill the gap where the flesh of my cheek should be. A networking of complex hooks and wires is clamped to the right side of my face. Only one half of the prosthesis has teeth, and it has a palatal arch and roof of the mouth.

During one of my visits to Manhattan from the hospital, I

went to an ophthalmologist who took a needle through the
near corner of my eye and shoved it through into my mouth
because my eye was sore and tearing and the tear duct had
been destroyed in surgery. He was trying to recreate the tear
duct.

On that same visit to New York, an ear specialist examined
me and said that I needed a tube to be put into the eardrum so
that I could have restored hearing, but he didn't do it at that
time because the doctors felt that I had endured too much pain
and that it was too soon after my major surgery. And so that
procedure was put off until months later.

Another physician, whom I had known for many years before my surgery and who saw me shortly after surgery, was so
horrified at my appearance and my handicap that he exclaimed
without thinking: "You'll never be a doctor now!"

When I stopped in the office of a friend to show how much
I had improved, the secretary, who had known me for years,
seeing me for the first time since my surgery, cried out, "Oh,
my baby! My baby! What have they done to you!" She fell to
the floor and hugged me about my knees, crying. A difficult
moment, not the best medicine for a very sick person, but I
respected her honest compassion.

The emotional strain of my illness took its toll on Chit, too.
He neglected his studies during the long trips from Bethlehem
to New Haven, but he came to visit me every weekend. One
day he gave a lovely damascene heart necklace to me. And on
that day he helped Mom to take me for my very first walk down
the hall. Blood ran constantly down my nose, and he got a box
of tissues and gently wiped the blood away as we walked. He
told me how much he loved me and missed me and that he
knew I would be getting better soon. He assured me of his
constant prayers.

"You'll be looking pretty again before long, Bea," he said.
"And I love you no matter what."

But on the following evening he telephoned from Bethlehem

and berated me for his poor performance on an exam, his lack of time to study, and his exhaustion. I tried to react calmly, but this tirade proved too much for me in my weakened condition. Still hooked up to IV and NG (nasogastric) tubes, I collapsed. Nurses and doctors rushed into the room, greatly concerned.

Recovery from this episode was rapid, but my health was too precarious to take any chances. From then on, only my immediate family was allowed to visit.

Finally the longest three weeks of my life came to an end. Each day when Dr. Karik visited, I reminded him of his promise to do everything within his power to see that I would be back in school before the end of October. One morning when he came to my room, he stood just inside the door, his eyes twinkling. "How would you like to go back to Philadelphia?" he asked.

I was up at dawn the next morning. I wanted to leave the hospital as soon as possible. How long would it take me to catch up with my class? I wondered.

The wounded tissue inside my face changed shape almost daily as it healed. Would my prothesis hold up until I could get a permanent one made? How long would the temporary crowns on the right side of my face continue to support this flimsy piece of plastic with the four teeth and gums attached? What would I do if the prosthesis fell out and broke? It was clamped into my mouth so precariously. Nothing was holding it in place on the left side of my face.

*Stop worrying*, I scolded myself. Think of happy things! Chit! He'd phone and be so happy that I was home again. I'd be back to school in time to go to the class Halloween party, and I wouldn't have the worry of an operation hanging over me. That was over and done with. But would my classmate still want to take me to the party? He might back out of his invitation after he saw me. I thought of Sabrina. How happy she'd be to see me! It wouldn't matter to her what I looked like. I'd throw my arms about her great barrel-shaped chest and . . .

I had no way of knowing that tears were spilling down my face. My cheeks were numb.

"Beatrice, whatever's the matter? Why are you crying?" I had lost much of the hearing on the left side and hadn't heard Mom come into the room.

"Nothing." I managed a smile.

Mom walked over to my chair and reached for a tissue from the little box I carried in my hand. "Tell me, dear, what's wrong?" I saw her wiping the tears from my face.

"Oh, Mommy," I sobbed. I raised my arms toward her. She cradled me then, her cheek resting lightly upon the top of my head. I drew away and looked up at her. "It's Sabrina!" I wailed.

"Sabrina! What about Sabrina?"

"I'm jealous of her jaws. Oh, Mommy, she has such beautiful strong jaws!"

Pain swept across Mom's face for just a moment and then she did an unexpected thing. She fixed her gaze directly into mine, and holding both of my hands in her own, she laughed and laughed and laughed. And a moment later when the nurses stepped in to say good-bye, that's how they found both of us—laughing!

# Chapter Nine

DURING the year I was overcoming the trauma of my surgery, so many people touched my life with the gift of their kindness, concern, and giving.

One of my six-year classmates had a hobby of gourmet cooking and delighted in tempting the palates of his friends. When I finally returned to MCP, he visited Mom and me at my apartment several times a week for the first couple of months—usually on his way dashing from one place to the other or on his way hiking. He brought samples of his culinary skills to tempt my flagging appetite, and always soft foods that I could eat.

Another classmate took time away from her own studies to help me write up a chart for my nutrition course. And as soon as I was able to be up and about for a couple of hours, she invited me over to her apartment for a get-together with one or two other students. After dinner, she would drive me home. Sometimes she would invite Mom, too.

Students and professors from Lehigh University, including

many whom I had never met, rallied around me with offers of friendship. I could always count on mail from Lehigh to lift my spirits. More than ever I was proud to be a part of that school.

Some time later, when people read my story in Associated Press articles, letters poured in from California to Florida. Mostly strangers to me, these people nonetheless reached out in love to give of themselves, their thoughts, their prayers. All wanted to offer encouragement and to wish me well.

Some shared their own stories with me. Mom read and reread these to me many times. They inspired me to keep going. Indeed, they affected my life in two very special ways.

First, from these people I learned how true it is that "no man is an island." No matter how independent we may be, in times of terrible stress it is very important to know that others care. It is not necessary for them to become deeply involved with us or with our problems—even just a cheerful greeting will do wonders to lift another's sprit. When a person is ill or in distress, it helps so very much to know that the world can be very friendly and caring. From my own experience, I can think of no better tonic for a patient than to receive a continuing stream of cheerful mail.

Second, I felt a commitment to these wonderful people who had touched my life with their gift of kindness and concern. Each of them had expressed appreciation for my courage—and so many had terrible suffering of their own. But there had been something about my story which had moved them to forget about themselves, to express their thanks to *me* for not giving up. I, in turn, felt a deep gratitude to each of them for having written to me and for having perservered themselves. I knew that it was important to them that I keep on going, and I was determined not to let them down.

To each of the many, many people who wrote to me, I would once again like to say *Thank you and God bless you*.

In retrospect, the love and concern shown to me by my professor of Community and Preventive Medicine, Peggy Stiler, M.D., was the most moving of all. During the time that I was in the hospital, Dr. Stiler had been ill with a brain tumor, but she had made the effort to send a cheery note to me. After I returned to classes, one of the students told me about Dr. Stiler's surgery and said that the tumor had been completely removed, that she was doing fine. In reality, she was dying, but she never mentioned a word of her continuing fight with illness. I suppose that she wanted to spare me the worry and wanted to encourage me to use all of my strength toward my own recovery.

Dr. Stiler and I were not intimate friends, but we were kindred spirits. I like to think that had she lived, we would have continued to nurture our growing friendship. I had met her during my first few days of getting to know my way around the medical college. She had been sitting alone in the cafeteria the first day I met her, writing and going over some papers until I sat next to her. She had looked up then and smiled, putting her papers into a folder.

"I was just doing some writing," she said.

"What are you writing about?" I asked, interested.

"The second edition of my book. I must finish it." She had written a major text, *Epidemiology*. Later, when I became one of her students, she autographed a copy for me. We chatted together often after our first meeting, and some days she brought homemade cookies in a brown paper bag to share with me.

When I first returned to school after my surgery, I felt a warm hand touch my shoulder. I turned and saw Dr. Stiler. She was wearing a kerchief on her head and looked somewhat thinner. She hugged me and said warmly, "I'm so glad you're back. I missed you."

Toward the end of my junior year, our conversation centered around my graduation the following year. I invited her to attend, but she declined. "I'd love to," she said, "but I can't. I must go to Germany to spend a year on a special project."

"I'll be taking electives away in New York during the beginning of senior year, so I guess I won't see you," I said. "I'm really looking forward to it, a real adventure."

"I know you'll do well," she said. She reached into a small bag and pulled out two of her special cookies. "Have one."

As we munched our cookies, I studied her. She was no longer wearing her kerchief, and her brown hair had grown back. She was done with her radiation treatments, I thought. "I'm so glad that we're well now," I said. Two years had passed since our surgeries.

She smiled. "I'm so proud of you," she said, "the way you were able to return to school, overcome your cancer, and now just think! You'll be graduating soon!"

"I'm proud of you too," I said. "Your book is almost finished. I'll want an autographed copy of this one too."

She hesitated. "You already have an autographed copy of the first edition," she said, avoiding an answer to my request. And then we walked down the hall together for the very last time. When we neared the library, I hugged her, kissed her goodbye, and hurried off.

Two months later, while in New York doing a subinternship, I received a copy of my school newspaper. Dr. Stiler had died from a brain tumor while in Germany. Evidently she had been battling cancer the entire time that I thought she was well. No wonder she couldn't autograph the second edition of her book. She must have known that she wouldn't be alive. Yet, I thought, look how proud she was of me, how uplifting she had been. I remembered her encouraging smile the day I had given my first speech to the class after my surgery. Her moral support had provided me with strength when I had really needed it. I only wished that I could have given something to her. And yet, I thought, perhaps my survival had been gift enough.

# Chapter Ten

I CHOSE a soft lavender wool jumper and a long-sleeved white blouse with tiny bunches of lavender flowers for my first day back at medical school. My long, light brown hair fell in soft, unstructured waves about my face. Both my face and my eye were still too raw to allow much makeup, but with Mom's help, I applied what I could to the "good" side of my face.

Mom was my chauffeur, and we agreed that she would drop me off and then wait in the hospital parking lot to drive me home as soon as I became tired.

As I walked up the steps of Ann Preston Hall to the locker room, I intuitively sensed the institutional smell even though my olfactory sense had been damaged. Downstairs in the lecture hall, the biochemistry class assembled. My classmates greeted me casually. "Hello," they said, one after the other, as though they had been seeing me every day of the week. One of them walked over to where I sat and remarked, "You look svelte." Actually I had lost so much weight that the jumper I had bought only the week before now hung on me like a sack.

No one mentioned my surgery. I sat in the class for fifteen minutes, hoping that I would learn by osmosis. I couldn't hear well and my eyes refused to focus. By the time I reached Mom's car, my legs wobbled to the point of collapse.

The following day when I arrived at the Ann Preston Hall lower lobby, someone guided me toward a big streamer strung across the wall. I didn't want to tell anyone that I couldn't read it, so I was glad when I heard a classmate say, "It says, 'Welcome back, Beatrice!' "

I looked about me. As far as I could tell, the whole class was there welcoming me back. And there was a sheet cake and punch. This would be my first time eating or drinking in public since my operation. I was afraid, but I determined to try. I took little sips of the punch and tiny bites of the sheet cake. Then I tilted my head back, hoping that gravity would take over. But in spite of my efforts, much of the food spilled through my nostrils into a tissue. After several attempts, I thought I had done enough for a first try and I relaxed, happy to see the faces of all those I had missed so much while I had been away. Again, after fifteen minutes, I returned to the car. This time, and every day thereafter, a friend carried my books for me.

At home, I rested for a short time and then insisted that Mom drive me back to school. Each day after that I tried to increase my endurance. I felt that that way I wasn't giving in.

I juggled my course schedule to get relatively easy courses out of the way, and I opted to take biochemistry-physiology during the coming summer. That first semester I took genetics, statistics, gross anatomy, psychiatry I, and nutrition. Mom read all my assignments to me, because I had trouble focusing my vision during that first year. Fortunately, medical students don't see patients until the end of the second year; training is based in textbooks and lectures for the first year and a half. With hard work, I was able to keep up with the pace.

Torturous medical school examinations were given to me orally, because I couldn't focus to write for any length of time. When I had to take written exams, I was permitted extra time.

Subsequently, I gave up vacations to catch up with missed courses. A friend helped me to write the nutrition log, where you tally up daily calories, intake and output.

A few days after I returned to school, a classmate wrote a song and dedicated it to me. At the end of the song he included a note:

> Beatrice,
> You are a very special person in so many ways. You have the "chutzpah" to keep going when so many of us would have long ago stopped. This song is dedicated to you, the Noble Crusader, from the MCP Class of '84.

That song, framed, hung in my bedroom through the four years of medical school. Often, when no one was near me and I did "feel so all alone," the love in that message helped to pull me through.

I waited each day for Chit to phone, but I didn't hear from him for several days after I left the hospital. Finally one evening he called.

"Hello, Bea."

"Chit! You finally called! Why didn't you call sooner?"

"I couldn't call you. I have a fifty-two-dollar telephone bill from last month, and then it cost a lot to travel to see you."

"Why didn't you write to me, then?"

"Why didn't you write to *me*?"

"I can't write. You know that. I can't see."

"If you can't see, you would be bumping into walls."

"That's a terrible thing to say. I can't believe you're saying that! There's a difference, you know, between not being able to see well enough to read and write, and bumping into walls."

"Well, I worried about you and I was waiting for you to call me. I'm always doing things for you. Why don't you think of me for a change?"

"You didn't even send me flowers when I was in the hospital."

"I bought you a gift, didn't I?"

"Yes, but the thing I really wanted was flowers. I asked you to get flowers—even a little bouquet or an African violet. Why wouldn't you do that?"

"You're spoiled. What did I get out of visiting you? What have you done for me lately?"

From then on, our relationship deteriorated. He telephoned many times and wanted to visit me, and he wrote many letters to me. He had a florist deliver a beautiful chrysanthemum plant with rust-colored blooms. *I didn't expect him to spend money for a fancy plant,* I thought. *Why couldn't he have given me even a single flower when I had asked for it in the hospital?* I buried my face in the flowers and cried. I missed him so! But I wasn't physically or emotionally able to cope with our many little bickerings, and so I distanced myself from him.

Early one morning during a class break as I was leaving to go home, my classmate reminded me that he would be taking me to the class Halloween party that evening. It would be held in a sorority house near my apartment, so I wouldn't have far to travel. And he understood that I would be able to stay at the party with him for only a few minutes.

I rested that afternoon and then dressed in a long white Mexican dress embroidered with big red and blue flowers at the neckline. And I wore a crazy green straw hat banded with multicolored flowers from an Acapulco trip. I couldn't wear a mask, because I couldn't touch anything to my face. My friend arrived, an excited, happy pirate, complete with paper sword, kerchief tied about his forehead buccaneer-style, and painted tattoos. I stayed at the party for less than half an hour, and then Mom came for me and drove me home. My friend walked me to the car, and some of my other classmates came outside and waved good-bye to me. When I got back to my apartment, Mom helped me undress and get into bed. I was so weak from the extra exertion that I could barely stand. But I was happy. I'd done something a little extra. I'd taken another step forward.

Simultaneously with my return to medical school, I had to

cope with countless visits to eye doctors, ear doctors, and dentists. My eyelid drooped, and the cornea was exposed to air more than usual, leaving the eye sore and dry. My eardrum was punctured and a tube inserted to improve my impaired hearing. Mom drove me to Manhattan and Connecticut for treatments and checkups.

Dental opinions differed as to the best way to handle my problem, and no one seemed able to offer a promising solution. Some of the dentists were argumentative and refused to even schedule me for appointments, saying that my treatment would take up too much of their time. They were totally indifferent to my plight. They had no interest in my determination to continue with my class. Rather, they insisted that if they were to care for me, I should give up medical school or at least defer it for one or two years.

I was beginning to feel completely alone, isolated in my dilemma. But during all of this time I never ceased to trust in God. Mom read portions of the Bible to me daily, and we did our best to center our minds in Him. When by the middle of November I was still without a suitable prosthodontist to reconstruct my face and mouth, Mom phoned the chief of dentistry at the University of Pennsylvania. He recommended Dr. Bal Singh.

Dr. Singh agreed to see me that Saturday morning for an evaluation. I liked him instantly. A quiet, soft-spoken Indian gentleman, he greeted us with interest and courtesy. As he examined me, his face showed none of the tension I had seen on the faces of others we had consulted. Neither did he exhibit an air of false confidence. He discussed his background and experience in the prosthodontic field and the problems peculiar to my case. His empathy was apparent.

He selected a team of dentists to coordinate my care under his supervision. Before a permanent prosthesis could be constructed, special crowns would have to be made, and a periodontist would have to cut away some of my gum and enlongate my remaining teeth. The temporary prosthesis that had been fitted during my stay in the hospital had become too loose, and it slipped down every time I opened my mouth. Whenever I smiled, my teeth bobbed up and down. So Dr. Singh designed another temporary prosthesis for me, and all of us prayed that it would last until the permanent one could be constructed.

I visited dentists several times a week for appointments that lasted up to eight hours. I went to classes for three hours in the morning, then to a dentist for seven or eight hours, then back to school for three hours of independent study in the medical library or the lab.

During the hours that the dentists worked on me, I wondered about my own reconstruction. How will this prosthesis compare to my natural mouth? How will it affect my image? Will I be able to kiss again, eat without pain, speak to groups of people, feel whole?

It's amazing, I thought, that people are born into this world with bodies equipped for survival. I prayed to God to be with me, and He was, every step of the way.

Often adjustments had to be made after my teeth were filed down. The bridge would be removed and my stubs exposed. The cool air, hitting my nerve endings, felt like electric shocks in my head. Dr. Singh continued to devote his Saturday mornings to me in order to fit me with a prosthesis that would fit the contours and the wire grooving in my mouth. Intermittently I visited the crown specialist. Each change affected the fit and the function of the temporary prosthesis. I presented a terrible challenge to Dr. Singh, but he never once allowed himself to become discouraged. Mom accompanied me to his office and sat in the room with me while he worked.

But at the other dentists' offices, pretty young nurses assisted the dentists, and in their presence I felt more mutilated than ever. Without a palate, without the upper left quadrant of my mouth, unable to speak, only stubs remaining of my filed-down teeth, my roots exposed and tender from all of the surgery, I felt a captive while molds and castings were made, plans set into motion. The pain was so tremendous that an anesthesiologist called in to control the pain gave me twenty injections with no relief.

It seemed as though all of my efforts to become whole again were futile. Inside myself I felt weary and distraught. *Perhaps God has changed His plans for me,* I thought as I prayed: "Not my will, but Thy will be done." I thought of 2 Samuel 22:7: "In my distress I called upon the LORD, and cried to my God: and he did hear my voice out of his temple, and my cry *did enter* into his ears."

On December 10, Mom's birthday, Dr. Stern gave me six tickets to see the Philadelphia 76ers at the stadium. I took Mom and four classmates. We had a great time, and after the game, returned to my apartment for wine and cheese, coffee and cake. Mary, my neighbor, joined us for refreshments. I felt recharged with new determination to keep on going.

When my friends volunteered to sing Christmas carols to the patients of the Medical College of Pennsylvania, I volunteered too. Early that evening, we went from room to room spreading cheer and goodwill. Our efforts were warmly received. At the door to one room I lingered behind the others. I was feeling tired and thought that perhaps I'd been pushing myself too much. *I think I'll go home now,* I thought. And then I saw that the patient we had thought asleep was sobbing, her arm thrown across her eyes, her hands clenching and unclenching in a gesture of despair. I walked into her single-bedded room and looked down at her without speaking.

She looked up at me, embarrassed. "You wouldn't know how I feel," she said defensively.

"Perhaps I would," I said quietly. "Tell me about it."

"I'm going to die." She watched me closely to see if the mention of death would frighten me away.

I told her a little about myself and said that I'd come through. She was encouraged to know that I had endured and was impressed with how well I looked. And she also appreciated knowing that I understood her loneliness. She no longer felt

like an alien creature on a strange planet; she knew that someone nearby could identify with her feelings and had even experienced them herself.

Just before Christmas vacation I sat for my final exam in
psychiatry. Before leaving for surgery in October, I had attended all of the classes and had participated actively in all of
the class activities. During the exam, since I could not focus my
eyes well enough to read or write for more than a few minutes
at a time, I was given a little extra time on the written test.
When the results of the exam were in, I was thrilled to learn
that I had scored 89. Ninety was honors, but those students
who had scored 89 and who had participated in class were also
given honors. And so I rejoiced—it was a kind of milestone for
me. But then I was puzzled when I saw my grade: P. This was
a pass-fail honors course. I was certain that the P was a mistake, and that the professor really intended to grade me H.

"I didn't give you honors because you weren't in my class
half the time," I was told in response to my questioning.

"How could I be in class?" I said. "I was in the intensive care
unit. Before I went to the hospital, I had been in every class."

"That doesn't matter," the professor said. "The point is, you
weren't in my class. I'm worried about you adjusting after all
the gala is out of the picture. The world's not going to baby you
and give you what you don't deserve."

But I felt that I had deserved honors because it was given to
others with the same grade as mine, provided that they had
participated in class. As far as I was concerned, at that time,
this was just one more knife to shove me over the edge.

I cried all the way home that Christmas when Mom came to
pick me up. I hadn't wanted treatment different from any that
had been shown to the rest of my classmates. I felt crushed by
such a cold, callous attitude. The injustice and the lack of feeling ruined much of that Christmas vacation.

When I returned to school after Christmas, our EMS (Emergency Medical Services) class began. We used little manne-
quins that we called "Annie." They were made of plastic and

had blond hair to make them appear more lifelike. We learned the ABCs of life support—airway, breathing, circulation. We had to blow into the mannequin to expand her lungs. This was the first time that I realized I was different from others. I couldn't give mouth-to-mouth resuscitation because I couldn't blow. I was allowed to stay in the class and learn the techniques because I could instruct others even if I couldn't perform the service myself. I became certified in EMS Basic Life Support, and at the end of medical school, I was certified in Advanced Cardiac Life Support.

On January 8, 1981, a copy of a letter that Dr. George Green had written to Dean Shoeman was placed in my mailbox. It did much to lift my spirits, especially after the blow I had received from the psychiatry professor before Christmas.

> Dear Dean Shoeman:
>
> The purpose of this letter is to accord proper recognition to Beatrice Engstrand's recent performance in our Principles of Medical Research course. The level of her accomplishment was so outstanding that the faculty of our department felt that some form of special notice should be given to it. Although she did not qualify for an Honors grade, we feel that the unique form of excellence which Beatrice displayed should not go unrecognized.
>
> We all are aware of the extreme personal hardship which Beatrice experienced this past semester and of the limitations which this placed on her participation in medical school activities. What is remarkable is that she was able to apply herself with such dedication, vigor, and ability to those tasks to which she was able to return—including our course. After being forced to miss several weeks of this course, she returned and, in spite of continuing physical difficulties, applied herself to making up the material she missed, including several assignments we agreed not to require of her.
>
> Beatrice set a personal goal for herself of earning Honors in the course, and in spite of the fact that I don't think the

learning of statistics comes easily to her, she almost achieved this goal—missing the cutoff by only a couple of points. We considered granting her an Honors grade anyway, in recognition of her special situation, but we decided that she really deserved more than the creation of a special category.

The faculty of this department have been deeply impressed by Beatrice's inspiring performance and by her spirit and character. We have been moved to do our part in according recognition to her and trust that this recognition will receive wider notice.

I learned from all of this that it's not the grades in themselves that are important. It's knowing deep down in your heart that you have done the very best that you could have done. And it's knowing that someone cares about you, that someone recognizes and appreciates your efforts. And it's a wonderful thing when you are treated with fairness. And I learned an even more important lesson from this experience: The world won't always treat you fairly. Be happy when it does. Be unshaken when it doesn't. And keep on persevering!

# Chapter Eleven

GROSS ANATOMY was the first course that I was able to take full-time after surgery. Each of us braced ourselves for the first day of this class. We would be facing a cadaver for the first time.

I followed the others into the anatomy room. Each of us drew upon our individual inner strength, independent of any other person. As we walked into the room, I saw twenty to thirty steel tables, stretcher-length, with big white plastic bags lying straight out on top. The bags were filled with formaldehyde and cadavers. The formaldehyde burned my nostrils. Everyone fell into a kind of stunned silence, and I felt an overwhelming sense of moroseness.

We were divided into small groups, and each group was assigned a cadaver. Each of us put on a long white coat and plastic gloves. My team was assigned to a short, middle-aged, stout black woman. Some others got young, skinny cadavers. They were all ages, and it was not a pleasant experience.

Once we were all assembled, we were told to take the body out of the bag and to shave all of the body hair except the hair on the head. We used soap and water to clean the body. Each of us had brought our own surgical equipment, which included a scalpel for cutting. This had a change of blades, because the blade dulls with use and must be changed like a razor blade.

When you first begin to dissect the cadaver, you do it in sections of body systems: head, arms, legs, abdomen, pelvis, not necessarily in that order. It is considered harder to work on the face and hands, because the face is intricately tied in with the identity of the person. And the human animal is the only one with a hand. When you dissect the hand of a person, you realize that you are working on a human. The same thing holds true for the face. It knocks your denial ability down.

During all of this time, my painful medical and dental visits continued as before, and I still had no permanent prosthesis. Many times I was tempted to give up and to stop trying.

But then a new turn of events came into my life. I began receiving letters from people who had severe illness or trouble. And people I would meet only casually would confide their troubles to me. They would tell me how my courage had been of help to them in their darkest hour or how my victory had given them the courage to keep going. One letter in particular really touched me. It was from a young woman whom I knew only casually.

> . . . Because of you I was able to find myself and my own strength. You see, not too long ago my husband lost his job. . . . Therefore we also lost our home. We had to live with friends and I had to divide my children. I kept the two youngest and my mom kept my two oldest. I was also in the hospital. . . . There were many things that happened during this period of time and I sort of gave up! Then I looked at all the things that you have been through and the way that you just kept going and you gave me courage. . . .

I didn't realize it all at once, but as letters continued to reach me, I began to realize that I could use my illness and the spiritual strength that God had given me to inspire others and to give them something to hang on to in their darkest moments.

There were many fears that I had to overcome. But the main thing I have learned is not to accept defeat and not to be ashamed of fear. Work to find ways to overcome the negatives.

For instance, I had never before feared walking in the snow or on icy sidewalks. But now I realized that if I slipped and fell, my prosthesis would become dislodged. If it fell and broke, it would take many months to have a new one constructed. And these would be months of agony in which I would not be able to function. And so I learned to exercise extra precaution on slippery surfaces and to wear rubber-soled flat boots when I had to walk in those conditions. I carried dress shoes with me to put on when I arrived safely at my destination. Eventually my tissues stabilized to the point at which it was possible to have two prostheses constructed, one as a spare.

Then, too, I feared driving a small car because any collision might have a greater impact than the same collision in a large car. At first, giving in to my fear, I purchased a very large car. Now I have come to a sensible compromise and drive a medium-size car.

Fear of mugging heightened almost to a state of panic. If I were to be struck on the head or on the side of my face, my prosthesis would dislodge and I couldn't scream for help or even speak to my attacker. I have overcome this fear by training myself to remain alert and to exercise reasonable caution. I progressed to the point where I was able to enjoy working as a resident at Kings County Hospital in Brooklyn.

I enjoy travel and flying, but after surgery, flying occasioned severe pain for me. My sinuses had been removed during surgery, and I have no way to adjust to the drastic change of altitude. Even a pressurized cabin does not protect me from this. At first I feared that I would no longer be able to fly. And then I found that medication can help to some extent. Through experimenting with several different approaches to this problem, I have overcome my fear and can once again enrich my life with travel.

Public speaking was another hurdle that I felt I must conquer, but I knew that it would take not only practice but guts. If I tried to deliver a talk and failed, I would be exposing myself as less than normal in yet another way, and for a long time I was afraid to try.

And then one day in my preventive medicine class I volunteered to prepare a speech on geriatrics. I selected Poppy as my example, and alone in the bedroom of my apartment, I practiced. At first it seemed as if I would never be able to project my voice loud enough to be heard in an auditorium. Then, too, when I tried to project, I had to take special care that my prosthesis didn't fall out and create an embarrassment. Fear took hold of me and I asked myself all kinds of negative questions: How could I manage to project? And if I did manage to project, how could I speak convincingly? How could I really concentrate on the content of my speech rather than on the mechanics of my mouth? But I was determined to try.

I didn't tell anyone how scared I was or how much it meant to me to be able to give this speech. Finally the day came, and I stood in front of a large auditorium filled with fellow classmates and several professors. As I approached the platform, I felt my heart pound, and my palms became sweaty. Pressure began building up in my body, and I began to tremble. How would I sound speaking with a mouth not my own? Would I make squeaking noises, or would I sound too nasal? Would they be able to hear me? Would I be able to enunciate well enough for them to understand what I was saying?

I looked around the room. All eyes were fixed upon me. There was absolute silence. Everyone was waiting to hear what I had to say.

Somehow I opened my mouth and began to speak. To my great relief, no one laughed at me. No one seemed aware of my inner struggle. Dr. Stiler, my professor and the director of the course, nodded with approval. Her eyes sparkled and her face was lit with enthusiasm. I knew that she was rooting for me.

After the speech, I received a standing ovation. My presentation had gripped the audience. During the class discussion that followed, it was unanimously agreed that I had captured the struggles of the geriatric population with great warmth and understanding.

That was another new beginning for me. After that I continued to address groups whenever the opportunity arose.

Human sexuality, legal medicine, oncology, death and dying, microanatomy, neurosciences, medicine and philosophy filled my second semester. My vision gradually improved, and I was now able to do my own reading and to drive my car. I reached out to embrace all of the life about me. And every day I thanked God for sparing my life and allowing me to be of service to my fellow man.

Philadelphia has good theater, and I made it a point to see several productions that year. I joined the AMA and enrolled in extra courses at school in order to become a Humanities Scholar upon graduation.

On April 13, 1981, I went to the Academy of Music to attend the inauguration of Maurice C. Clifford, M.D., seventeenth president of the Medical College of Pennsylvania. As I watched Dr. Clifford walk down the long aisle toward the podium, in the company of his distinguished peers, I was impressed by the aura of friendly dignity that emanated from him. *As a black man, he must have had many obstacles to overcome, many prejudices to surmount*, I thought.

His inaugural address inspired me, and I listened attentively to every word. I felt proud to have him as the president of my medical college, and everything he said had a truthful and sincere ring to it. His creed paralleled my own.

I believe in the family . . . natural and honorary . . .
friends dear as kin. . . .
I believe that since we survive our newborn helplessness

only through the gift of loving care, that gift endows each
of us with something to give back.

I believe in prayer, and I believe that however we pray,
our good Father returns His own good and timely answer.


*What a great human being! What a great president he will be,* I
thought. I wrote to him expressing my thoughts. And to my
delight, he replied.

Some time later when I finally met Dr. Clifford personally, I
found him to be all of the things that I had imagined he would
be—warm, friendly, caring, and dignified. His office typified
the qualities of the man—warm, homey, elegant in the tradi-
tion of the MCP spirit. And a big grandfather clock made it all
just perfect. In the few minutes that we spent together, we
instantly felt a warm friendship.

Neither of us mentioned my illness. Instead, we spoke of
mutual interests. After that meeting I realized that this had
been the first time since my surgery that someone had talked to
me without making some remark about my illness, even if only
to express sympathy and concern. That meeting represented a
milestone to me! Someone had been able to talk with me and to
ignore my disfigurement!

When I mentioned my desire to write about humanistic issues, Dr. Clifford suggested that I contact Nancy Koppel, the
director of publications for MCP. And so it was through Dr.
Clifford's encouragement that I developed my interest in writing. Eventually I wrote columns for the MCP publications, including two viewpoint columns for *MCP Today*.

However, it seemed that each time I achieved a degree of
normality, something happened to remind me of my extreme
vulnerability. One morning my crowns fell out in my apartment as I was getting ready to leave for school. Of course, my
prosthesis came out too. In pain and unable to speak, I drove
to downtown Philadelphia and waited outside the dentist's
office until it opened.

Another time, I went to the Thousand Islands for a few days' vacation. Before leaving Philadelphia, I had gone to Dr. Singh so that he could check my prosthesis. He made a minor adjustment, but after several days the adjustment had caused an ulcer in my mouth and I had to cut my vacation short. It seemed that I would never be able to think of myself as normal. And so I determined to think of the happy things in life and to weed out the negatives whenever possible.

I have learned that when you have a multitude of problems, it is neither necessary nor wise to attempt to tackle them all at once. Tackle and overcome them one by one. If you should happen to choose one that proves too difficult for you to handle at once, set that particular problem aside for the time being and tackle a smaller, easier-to-handle problem.

After that, gradually go back to the original problem that stumped you. You will find that you will have learned to cope by doing. You will have become more resilient, stronger. And this newfound strength within you will carry you over the rough spots.

It's not an easy road. But why should it be? Even so-called normal people who don't suffer from handicaps have many other problems with which to contend. No two people are alike. The same handicap can present completely different problems to different persons. What may seem to be the greatest of problems to one person may appear to be the least cause of concern to another.

But all people with handicaps do face extra challenges, additional obstacles. A prime goal is to remain strong. If you sink down into defeat and into despair once in a while, pull yourself out of it. Don't stay there. Wallowing in mud is for pigs, not people.

You are God's person. Your body is a vehicle for your soul and your personality. Treat it well and respect its needs. But if it should become damaged, your personality and your soul-power can still remain intact if you will allow them to. Let your light shine, as the Bible says. No one can do this better than you. How many so-called normal people waste their lives by being grumpy, greedy, groaning!

Your gift of spirit can be shared with others in many ways. There is so much unhappiness in the world that people flock to a happy person, a confident person, a secure person. Regardless of handicaps, that person will attract others, because everyone wants to be near happy people. That kind of spirit radiates and is tonic for those it touches.

When I was a little girl, I used to hear my grandfather Poppy quote an old saying, "Build a better mousetrap and the world will beat a path to your door." Well, if you keep your light shining, you will have built a happy, harmonious spirit, and those who hear of you will beat a path to your door. In giving joy and strength to others, your light will reflect back onto your own life.

# Chapter Twelve

SOPHOMORE YEAR in medical school was the turning point in my life. During that year I became trapped in a depression more dreadful, more terrifying, than anything I had ever known. Before I conquered it, it threatened to wipe out all the progress that I had made. It became a terrorizing force that seemed to control every moment of my life, night and day. It drove me almost to the point of suicide.

There were many reasons for my depression. Almost one full year after surgery, I was still not put together well. My physical complaints seemed endless.

Ugly brown scabs continued to form all along the surgery site. Sometimes these would be one inch, sometimes two inches, in length. And there were many of them. At first the surgeon picked them away. Gradually I learned to use long, slender tweezers and reach up into the cavity to extract them.

My nose chapped constantly. Fluid continued to spill out of it after eating and drinking, because we hadn't been able to get a tight seal with my prosthesis. At the end of each day, I had emptied a full box of tissues.

I became a living barometer. Rain, storms, humidity, any changes in the weather, gave me severe headaches and pain. I wore a scarf to protect my cornea from cold and wind. On the other hand, heat made my tissues swell. My air conditioner operated year-round.

Impaired hearing made it impossible for me either to use a telephone with my left ear or to hear anything being said from my left side.

My numb left cheek developed an itch that no amount of scratching could relieve.

An ache deep down in the bones of my legs, feet, and arms became so severe that at times I could barely stand. For relief when I went to bed at night, I turned on my air conditioner, used an electric heating blanket, and wrapped electric heating pads about my legs.

Only one side of my mouth could eat, chew, or taste. Even on that side, the sense of taste was diminished. I couldn't bite into an apple or chew gum or eat anything but soft foods and tiny, bite-sized pieces of fork-tender meat. Immediately after eating, my mouth and cavity had to be irrigated with a syringe, and my prosthesis had to be removed for cleaning. Without this cleaning, unbearable pressure built up to the orbit of my eye. Even with this cleaning, my remaining tissues and gums were irritated and inflamed.

I lived in constant fear of losing my remaining teeth. Without them, there would be no support for a prosthesis.

In addition to all of these things, I also had to cope with facial disfigurement.

With these problems piled one on top of the other, when depression attacked I didn't understand what was happening to me. It seemed as if my emotions belonged to someone else, as if I were skimming by on the edge of my life, not really a part of it.

At the end of freshman year, I had stayed at my apartment in Philadelphia and had mapped out a self-study plan for biochemistry-physiology, a fourteen-credit course. I had passed the final exam and was once again on a par with my class.

But at the end of the summer, when my classmates returned to school refreshed, I felt drained. It was the first time in my life that I couldn't work up any enthusiasm about starting a new school year.

I experienced feelings of isolation and loneliness even though people were around me. Once in a while my classmates talked with me about their future plans, but no one asked me about mine. It seemed as if I wasn't expected to have any. I listened attentively while one student talked about becoming an air force physician. Both the navy and the air force had attempted to recruit me prior to my surgery. At one time I had even toyed with the idea of becoming a space physician. Now those options were closed to me.

I tried to fill my mind with positive thoughts, but nothing helped. Insomnia took over my nights, and I walked into classes without sleep.

And then one day in psychiatry, the professor talked about depression, and I identified my problem. I was in a state of deep depression. My depression wasn't obvious. I kept a cheerful appearance, but I knew that I was losing control. I wanted to reach out for help to the psychiatrists at school, but I couldn't see my way through the maze to approach one of them. I felt like a juggler—as if I were throwing all the balls up in the air at once and something was bound to fall.

That something was pathology. It was my most vulnerable spot, because the professor seemed to go out of his way to make things difficult for me. Some of our tests were hours long, and during short class breaks I ate snacks in order to keep up my energy. I had been diagnosed as having hypoglycemia (low blood sugar). When I asked permission to go to the ladies' room so that I might clean my mouth after eating, the professor refused. He didn't even try to understand my plight, although he was an oral surgeon as well as a pathologist.

"You can clean your mouth here in class," he said.

Of course, this was impossible. I wouldn't remove my prosthesis and syringe the cavity without absolute privacy.

That night in my apartment, unable to find any way out of my plight, I cried for hours. During that semester, my weight zoomed out of control and I gained twenty pounds.

After that, I didn't eat during class breaks, and of course, I couldn't function well. Desperate, I requested tutoring. My professor assured me that tutoring was not available. "You should never have returned to school," he said. He seemed to resent the fact that I hadn't stayed behind a year. Later, I found out that several students had been tutored by another physician in the department.

Just before the pathology midterm, as the exam was being distributed, a professor who had drawn my blood the week before informed me that my liver enzymes were highly elevated and that the results were consistent with metastatic liver disease.

My world bottomed out. I said, "What do I do now?"

She said that she wasn't 100 percent sure. To be sure, she said, she needed to run more tests—that the only other thing it could be was hepatitis.

I failed the midterm and went to her for further testing. A diagnosis was made of non-A non-B hepatitis—a result of contaminated blood I had received during the second surgery. I failed pathology, but I was permitted to advance to the second semester of the year. Again I would have to spend another summer vacation at school—this time in order to pass pathology.

Thoughts of suicide crept into my thinking. I willed these thoughts out of my mind. Yet, in spite of my best efforts, they kept coming back stronger. It seemed that one part of me, out of control, wanted to die. But the conscious part of me that I controlled wanted to live. I felt torn between the two. I didn't know which part of me would win. And I was frightened.

My prayer became an urgent plea: "God! Help me!" I repeated the Lord's Prayer many times a day. Whenever I felt

completely overwhelmed, I said, "Thy will be done," and re-
lied on Him to see me through. Always, I kept two verses in my
heart: "He restoreth my soul . . . Yea, though I walk through
the valley of the shadow of death, I will fear no evil: for thou *art*
with me; thy rod and thy staff they comfort me." (Psalm 23:
3–4)

And then God answered my prayer.

As I contemplated my situation, I suddenly became angry. I
became angry about failing pathology. I became angry about all
the unfair things that had happened to me. I became angry at
the cancer. I became angry about all the physical ailments that
were trying to defeat me after I had fought so hard.

I realized that I could quit and feel sorry for myself, or I could
persevere and experience the best of life. I decided to concentrate on the present moment and give each task my best effort.
As I began to take active steps in every area of my life, I found
much strength inside myself.

Painful, depressing dental visits became bearable when I associated them with other things. I did not become as depressed
when I would do something I enjoyed the same day—activities
as simple as shopping, taking a walk in the park, or dining at
a good restaurant. I might buy a bar of fragrant soap in a pretty
wrapper or go to a nearby bakery for coffee and a croissant.
Those diversions provided time for meditation, and I soon realized what good company I could be to myself.

I cast out false pride and reached out to others for help. Some
areas of physiology were fuzzy to me, because I had missed so
many lectures during my freshman year. Introduction to Physical Diagnosis, my first exposure to patients, was about to begin, and I wanted to do well in it. I went to Dr. Lawrence
Feldman, professor and director of the course, and asked for
help. I told him that I had failed pathology and that if I should
fail another course, I would have to repeat the year. Dr. Feldman immediately telephoned Dr. Nancy Griffiths, a young,
brilliant clinician. With her help, I quickly caught up with my
studies.

Depression hung on like a pit bull, but I believed that it was losing ground, because I was now able to study and to concentrate. Day after day I made a conscious effort to accept myself. Before, if I had been hurt, I healed. I pictured myself like a child who scrapes a knee and has a mother bandage it; when the dressing is removed, the knee is healed. Days, months, a year, drifted by before I accepted the fact that this change would indeed be permanent.

Finally I accepted myself with limitations *and* potentials and set out each day to enrich my life and the lives of others.

I chaired a conference on the role of handicapped physicians.

I wrote columns and articles for MCP publications.

I accepted an invitation to speak at Lehigh University in a panel discussion for the health professions.

"Uncle Bunny" and I performed ventriloquism and made balloon animals at the annual Christmas party for pediatric patients at MCP and for the reunion luncheon of MCP "graduates" of the neonatal intensive care unit. At the request of Dr. Robert Snow, pediatric neurologist, Mom and I performed for the handicapped and crippled children at the Blythedale Children's Hospital in Valhalla, New York.

And then one day, during prayer, an inspiration came to me! I would combine the power of prayer, positive thinking, and self-imaging to improve my appearance. My parents had been married in the Marble Collegiate Church on Fifth Avenue and Twenty-ninth Street in New York City when Dr. Norman Vincent Peale was the pastor. When I was a young girl, Mom had given me a copy of Dr. Peale's book, *The Power of Positive Thinking*. Every so often I would open it, read a few sentences, and place it back on the shelf. Now I determined to read it daily, together with my Bible.

I thought of my face and meditated. "He hath made every *thing* beautiful in his time. . . . I know that, whatsoever God doeth, it shall be for ever: nothing can be put to it, nor any thing taken from it. . . . That which hath been is now; and that which is to be hath already been. . . ." (Ecclesiastes 3: 11, 14–15)

The importance of self-imaging cannot be stressed too much. Your appearance to the outer world is reflected in the way you think. Your mind helps to shape your body, and your mind helps to shape your world.

*The Power of Positive Thinking* says:

To change your circumstances, first start thinking differently. Do not passively accept unsatisfactory circumstances, but form a picture in your mind of circumstances as they should be. Hold that picture, develop it firmly in all details, believe in it, pray about it, work at it, and you can actualize it according to that mental image.

The major thrust of medical and dental efforts in my case was directed toward refashioning what remained of the inside of my face in order to construct a functional, less-irritating prosthesis. Hopefully, this would enable me to present myself to others in an aesthetically pleasing manner. Reconstruction meant cutting millimeters of remaining gum tissue, root canal work, filing down and capping of remaining teeth. These procedures required great skill, patience, and innovation on the part of the practitioners, because they were working on severely traumatized tissues. I had had skin grafting on the *inside* of my cheek, and grafted skin is not strong enough to support bone transplants. And my medical team had determined to leave my defect uncovered in order to detect any sign of recurring cancer or tissue changes.

Many people wrote to me after seeing my picture in newspapers or on the cover of the *Lehigh Alumni Bulletin*, fall 1985. They said that they looked forward to the time when they, too, could have such excellent plastic surgery. But the truth is that I have not had any plastic surgery on the outside of my face. Prayer, positive thinking, and self-imaging—along with prosthetic reconstruction and an excellent surgeon—helped to recontour my face, and against all odds, made me an attractive person once again.

* * *

Toward the end of the second year at medical school, our class was divided into teams, and we had our first exposure to patients. My team consisted of myself and two male students. We wore white coats for the first time, and we carried black doctor's bags with medical instruments inside. My team was sent to the VA Hospital in Philadelphia. Medical staff asked the patients for permission to have students interview them and take their histories. Then Dr. Feldman handed each team an outline of questions. We were to make a diagnosis from the answers. Holding the questions in one hand, we read them from the paper and then turned to ask the patient. We stumbled over medical charts that were like a foreign language to us. They had their own special shorthand: HA, headache; SX, symptoms. Our patient was amused by us, but cooperative. I think we were the highlight of his day!

Another day with the same team, I was performing a physical on a middle-aged man with severe aortic stenosis, a serious heart problem. He told us that he knew all about his condition. His physician had given him a diagram of his heart. He offered to explain this to me. As I continued with the physical, I began to comprehend that this man needed to understand all he could about his condition. He needed to feel that he had some control. And he preferred to view his problem as a scientific puzzle rather than as a life-threatening situation. As I listened to his heart, I thought that he might like to hear how his murmur sounded. Gently I placed the stethoscope's diaphragm over the base of his heart and instructed him to listen to the "whoosh." When he heard his murmur, his face flushed with excitement, like a child with a new toy. "That's wonderful!" he said. He flashed a broad smile at me. "I never knew it sounded like that. Thank you." I knew that it was more than listening to his heart that had thrilled this man; it was the empathy displayed for his particular needs.

Finally, there was the former merchant marine, a rugged, unshaven, intimidating man. He was lying in bed as I entered his room. When he heard me enter, he sat up and exclaimed in a gruff voice, "All right, interview me! But don't ask none of those personal questions." In subtle ways I let him realize that I respected him, his thoughts, and his experiences. I listened to him with interest. Sensing this, he no longer felt threatened by me, and his tone softened. "Listen to me," he said, mellowed. "People like to be treated by a doctor who really cares for them. I had a doctor once. I'll never forget. Every evening, after work, he came back to visit his patients for a few minutes just to talk about things in general. The guys really loved him."

As a medical student just starting to learn about clinical medicine, I was beginning to formulate my own perception of medicine and what type of physician I would strive to become. And I knew that I wanted to touch the lives of my patients by addressing them as people, not just as pathological entities.

Listening to the merchant marine, I vowed somehow to remain concerned with the patient as a human being, because to me, a blend of the two—humanistic and technical—is the highest form of the art of healing.

Now, as a resident neurologist at Downstate, I feel like a den mother to the medical students who live in my dorm building. One young student across the hall from me knocked at my door the other day. She was wearing her white coat and carrying her instruments for the first time. She had just seen her first patients.

"Did you test for *this*?" I asked.

"Oh, no! I forgot."

I, now a wise old owl, said, "Well! How do you expect to make a diagnosis?"

At the end of the second year of medical school, I passed Part I of the National Board examinations. I remained at my apartment in Philadelphia, preparing for the pathology exam. Two weeks before my repeat final, the bones in my legs became so painful that I found it difficult to stand. Dr. Karik, who continued to oversee my care, suggested a CAT scan. Naturally I was devastated. *I will take this test on schedule,* I thought. *I have stud-ied for it. I'm ready for it. Nothing will keep me from my goal.* ". . . Forgetting those things which are behind, and reaching forth unto those things which are before, I press toward the mark for the prize. . . ." (Philippians 3: 13–14) I took the final on schedule and passed.

My feet and legs continued to be painful, and at one point in my third year of medical college, I was unable to fit a shoe, a sneaker, or a slipper on my foot. The foot blew up like a bal-loon. I consulted an internist, an orthopedic specialist, a neu-rologist, a podiatrist, and a rheumatologist, all without relief. Finally a podiatrist lent me a special type of casing for my foot so that I could walk on it. I didn't tell any of my classmates or professors what I was suffering. I said that I had a piece of glass in my foot. When I improved enough to wear soft slippers, one professor wrote a criticism of me for wearing bedroom slippers on rounds. Dean Shoeman, who I am certain understood more than she let on, had the criticism withdrawn.

My depression was under control by now, and I was no longer filled with fear. When I went for a repeat body scan and chest X ray at Harkness Pavilion on December 27, 1982, I faced it with confidence. I knew that I had done all that I could do to right my life.

As a third-year student, I worked with residents and attend-ing physicians—rotating through surgery, medicine, neurol-ogy, psychiatry, obstetrics/gynecology, and pediatrics.

In my fourth year, I completed with honors a neurology ophthalmology elective at Wills Eye Hospital; a subinternship in neurology at Memorial Sloan-Kettering Cancer Center, Neu-rological Institute, and Columbia-Presbyterian Babies' Hospi-tal. I also did a gastroenterology elective at the New York Hospital–Cornell University Medical Center. I was privileged to present part of Grand Rounds on Lyme Disease at the Neuro Institute, and I felt right at home there. A large portrait of Dr. Glickmann, with whom I'd chatted often, hung in the lovely old library. Pediatric neurology at Babies' Hospital was a nostalgic elective for me too. I remembered how I had been a patient at Babies' Hospital when I had been a child, and I thought how far I had come. And I felt so grateful to all those who had helped me along my way.

One day, accompanied by a psychiatrist preceptor, I entered the room of a woman in the terminal stage of cancer. She felt tired and was reluctant to speak with me until I assured her that I would not take long, and that all I wanted to know is what brought her into the hospital. I remained silent while she rapidly conveyed her history to me. Her personality unfolded as she spoke, and she began to share her feelings with me. She conveyed sorrow at being unable to watch her grandchildren grow up, and at leaving her husband, her first lover, behind. She expressed her guilt for having cancer, her fear of death, her devout belief in God. She accepted her fate with strength, and the more she talked to me and voiced her concerns, the stronger she became. She began to speak with enthusiasm about a trip she would plan with her husband, about visiting her daughters. Even impending death was not going to destroy this woman's spark. As a medical student, I could not erase her destiny, yet I could listen while she told me her story. And at the end of the interview, I knew that she was focusing her thoughts upon the positive things that she would be doing with her family right up to the end of her life.

Another patient was a seventy-year-old man with a diagnosis of oat cell carcinoma with cerebral metastasis. Despite this man's seemingly hopeless condition, he continued to have an optimistic attitude toward life. Each morning as I entered his room before rounds, he would arouse himself eagerly, greet me with a smile, and voice few, if any, complaints.

I remember one morning in particular. He was sitting up in bed with his new prosthetic leg beside him. As I entered his room, I noticed he was staring out the window. His eyes seemed to rest upon an inconspicuous chapel nestled among the interlocking streets and row houses of East Falls. "You know," he said with pride, "my grandfather helped build that chapel. My family, they helped build these parts." Listening attentively as he disclosed his family history to me, I realized that he wanted me to know that he, too, formed part of that heritage. When he finished his tale, he questioned me, "Do you believe in God and life eternal?" With conviction, I answered affirmatively. Meekly he implored, "Will you pray for me?" I nodded. He clasped my hand, and with his eyes watering, he said, "As long as I live, I will always remember you."

In my death and dying course, we had often discussed issues related to care for the critically ill. We were made keenly aware of their needs, and we learned how important it is not to shun the dying nor to isolate them. They, too, need to feel a part of the world. This concept inspired me to spend extra time each day with my terminal patients. It also gave me courage to face the moment of death with a patient if the need should arise.

One particular night on call demanded such courage. Entering the room of a patient, I stood watching as my resident performed cardiopulmonary resuscitation. Only hours before, this patient had been telling my resident and me about her hopes of leaving the hospital and returning home.

Now, as she lay on her bed, her legs and arms outstretched, her EKG revealed no heartbeat. Lines were started, fluids pushed, medicines given. Doctors, nurses, aides, worked to restore her life. My resident, calm and composed, controlled the scene. The room portrayed a picture of life battling with death, medicine's ultimate challenge.

It was the first time I had witnessed a person's demise. All that remained when the code cards were withdrawn was a lifeless corpse who, a short time before, had been a vibrant being with life and dreams like the rest of us.

One night I was called upon to draw blood on a stroke patient. As I entered the room, I noticed that he was contorted out of shape, motionless in his bed. I recalled the times we had discussed that no matter how ill or unresponsive a patient

might seem, he might still be aware of the actions and conversations around him. Taking advantage of that lesson, I proceeded to tell the patient that I was aware he was trying to
communicate with me, and that I understood how he must feel
locked within his body. I told him, however, that sometimes
stroke victims can recover some of their body's functions over
time, and that he must be patient. I also informed him that I
planned to pursue a neurological career and to dedicate my life
to helping people in his condition. I saw a tear form in his eye
when I finished speaking. But I was still not certain that he was
cognizant of anything that I had said.

A couple of weeks later, I was asked to draw blood on this
same patient. As I approached his bed, I saw that some motion
of his limbs had returned, and that some of his speech was
restored. When he saw me, his eyes lit up and he said, with
effort, "I heard what you said that other night."

And then there was the patient on my medical rotation whom
Dr. Griffiths thought was too difficult for a medical student to
manage. I often think of that patient now and of how happy
she would be to see how skilled I have become with blood
gases. A seventy-two-year-old woman, she had come to MCP
with a multitude of problems: heart failure, kidney failure, permanent valve replacements, frequent bouts with infections, in-
stalled pacemaker, occult lower GI bleed, obesity, diabetes,
rheumatic disease. Her oxygen status had to be monitored,
because she had a tracheostomy and pulmonary problems. I
was told to get blood gases on her.

Blood gases can be quite painful, and blood drawing was a
new technique for me. Every day I would tremble, shake, and
sweat, and every day she would growl at me through her tracheostomy site. She became a symbol to me of my own inad-
equacy. I saw her and I thought, *Blood gas!* She tried to
communicate to me, but because of her intubation, the only
sounds she could make were hisses and gurgles. Finally she
wrote a note and handed it to me: *I don't want you to draw my*

*blood*. She also refused to have an intern take her blood. The entire teaching team I was on started to dislike her, because it was our first experience with a noncompliant patient.

Dr. Griffiths spoke firmly to all of us. "If you can't do a good job, don't do it," she said. She explained that this was an old woman who, with her problems, probably did not have long to live and just didn't want to be made miserable. After that, I began to see the woman in a new light. From that moment on, I approached her with more understanding. And our relationship ran smoothly. Some time later, when I saw her on a readmission, she was so happy to see me that she held on to my hand. Dr. Griffiths was the one who told me of her death because she knew that the patient had become very fond of me. I had gotten to like her too. She was so spunky, and she'd been through so much. Knowing her not only helped me to forget myself in service to others, but also helped me to realize the importance of training new students and residents under me to do blood gases correctly and painlessly.

During all of this time my mouth tissues were still irritated, a cause of concern to both my surgeon and my prosthodontist. Dr. Jacob M. Stein of New York City, a world-renowned prosthodontist, dental surgeon, and crown specialist, agreed to examine my mouth. Dr. Stein, Dr. Karik, and Dr. Singh conferred, and Dr. Singh was happy to report that Dr. Stein might be able to improve the condition of my mouth by making a new prosthesis with specific changes. I was relieved, because I knew that I would be doing my internship and residency somewhere in New York, and it would be impossible for me to commute to Philadelphia for my care.

Dr. Stein had been the youngest major in the Dental Corps during World War II. Twenty-five years old, he had had a dental lab and clinic in Manila, where he had treated our GIs as well as General and Mrs. Douglas MacArthur. Although he was so young, Dr. Stein had gained technological know-how from working in his father's dental lab, the largest one in New

York at the time. His dad had named it Owl Dental Laboratory, because employees worked on shifts around the clock. After the war, Dr. Stein had taken postgraduate courses in New York University and then worked under Dr. John Convers, a plastic surgeon.

Both Dr. Stein and Dr. Singh are very devout men, and they practice their beliefs. Dr. Singh is a Hindu, and when I graduated from medical college, he and his wife gave me an original painting, framed, from India, of Lord Krishna and his beloved Radha and her friends. Dr. Stein tells me that he prays to God every day asking Him to strengthen his skills before he does his work with patients.

I asked Dr. Stein what particular case impressed him the most, and he mentioned two. The first had been a patient of Dr. Convers's—a young boy born with a severe cleft palate and cleft nose. His family had cast him into the jungles of Panama and left him to die. An American engineer found him and brought him back to New York for care. The *Reader's Digest* had carried the article.

The other case was of a Polish woman, a refugee from a German concentration camp. Still alive, she writes to Dr. Stein. He told me her story:

"Her face was crushed, almost unrecognizably, by the rifles of the keepers of the camp. One-half her jaw was removed. Her teeth were all out; her face was completely disfigured. She was scheduled to go into the gas chambers. Just at that moment, the Russians took over the camp and rescued her. But they didn't know what to do with her because she was unable to eat—her face was so disfigured—and she would have died. So they turned her over to the British, who turned her over to the Americans. It was then that she got under the care of Dr. Convers. Dr. Convers and I worked together on this lady, and it took us five years of intensive work to make her look normal."

Now that I have gotten to know Dr. Stein very well, I know that he is a man who likes to help people who have been hurt by situations beyond their control. His dream is to build a head-and-neck prosthodontic center where everything can be coordinated under one roof.

I don't know exactly when this happened, but some time shortly after my first meeting with Dr. Stein, my spirits lifted. My depression was completely gone. Now, once again, I was free to pursue my dream with a happy heart.

On Founder's Day I was completely surprised and thrilled when Dean Shoeman presented me with two awards: the Beatrice Sterling Hollander, M.D., WMC '41 Memorial Prize to the student in the graduating class who shows promise of leadership, high character, and creativity in her profession; and the Leopold Canales Award for excellence in neurology. I also graduated as a Humanities Scholar, and I had matched at North Shore University Hospital, Manhasset, New York, for internship and at The New York Hospital–Cornell University Medical Center in Manhattan for neurology residency.

My dream came true on May 30, 1984. Alongside my fellow six-year students from Lehigh, I received the M.D. degree from the Medical College of Pennsylvania. I've never been happier than that day in Philadelphia when the physician's tunic was placed upon my shoulders.

The Associated Press covered my story. One of their photographers and writers interviewed me and took pictures throughout the graduation ceremony. Leading newspapers picked up the story, and from all over the country, people wrote to express their love and their joy at my victory over cancer. I sincerely appreciated every letter, and I answered each one personally. One letter writer with whom I continue to correspond is a gentleman in his nineties who, a few years ago, had a radical maxillectomy. He lives in a Soldiers and Sailors Home in Pennsylvania and writes upbeat, chatty letters to me on his typewriter. A therapist helps him to make pictures and cards that he sends to me. Mom and I surprised him one day with a telephone call.

I hope that reading about my successful journey through severe depression will comfort and encourage others. If I did it, you can do it too. If you were about to take a journey into the jungles of the Amazon, across the desert, through the Himalayas, you would appreciate any guideposts along the way. And so it is with depression. There were ten steps that I took in my journey. At the time, I didn't realize that I was taking these steps. It seemed as if I were walking an uncharted course. But it wasn't uncharted at all. When I reached out in prayer and said, "Thy will be done," God guided me every step of the way.

These are the ten steps that I took. They helped me. I believe that they can help you too.

## *Journey Through Depression*

1. Identify the problem.
2. Hit bottom, but don't give up. Instead, become angry.
3. Recognize your need for help. Cast out false pride. Reach out to others for help, and *determine* to help yourself.
4. Be willing to *work* to conquer your problem. Take active steps in every area of your life.
5. *Be* what you *are*. Accept yourself with limitations *and* potentials, and set out each day to enrich your life and the lives of others.
6. Combine the power of prayer, positive thinking, and self-imaging. Replace negative thoughts with positive thoughts. No matter how bad you feel, just keep saturating your mind with positive thoughts. Eventually they will take hold. Read, watch, and listen to positive, happy things.
7. Forget self in service to others. Go one step beyond your own needs.

8. Persevere. Concentrate on the present moment and give each task your best effort.
9. Cast out fear. Do all that you can to right your life. Then relax and let God take over.
10. Live always with a dream. When you fulfill one dream, find another.

# Chapter Thirteen

AT THE END of medical school, newspaper headlines read: SHE BEATS PAIN TO BECOME A DOCTOR. Now I was about to reach for yet another dream—to become a neurologist. Neurology intrigues me as a field of medicine. In addition to dealing with the brain, it also draws into its realm many patients with chronic problems. Using my own suffering as a base, I felt that I could empathize with my patients and could offer enthusiastic support to them. I would encourage them to keep going in spite of limitations.

Neurology requires one year of internal medicine and three years of neurological training. For my first year of medicine I opted to go to North Shore University Hospital, a teaching center of Cornell University Medical College. While I was there, my supervised training included exposure to Memorial Sloan-Kettering Cancer Center, total patient care, both acute and chronic, and instruction in the performance of technical skills, such as arterial lines, Swan Ganz catheters, and central lines.

In a group of about thirty new interns, I was greeted early in

July 1984 by Patrick Segan, M.D., director, Department of Medicine; Samuel Fry, M.D., associate director; and Jack Houston, Graduate Training Programs director, as well as by many other staff physicians and residents. My fellow interns and I did not know then that we were about to enter a world unlike any other we had ever known. This would be a world of thirty-six-hour work shifts every three days, one complete day off a month, life and death decisions, demanding academic testing, and little, if any, free time.

I had come to North Shore thinking that it would be clean, easier than an inner-city hospital for the dreaded internship year, and I looked forward also to returning to Long Island from Philadelphia. I had been away six years. Little did I know that I'd have so little time to myself.

Only after one successfully struggles through the hazing of internship can one appreciate it. The rigors of internship shape your future practices as a physician by providing a groundwork where the technical, academic, and humanist merge.

I had been placed in the CCU (coronary care unit) to work the first month of my medical internship year, notorious July. The CCU consisted of four beds with monitors. These beds were usually occupied by patients with new MIs (myocardial infarction, or heart attack) who came into the emergency room complaining of chest pain, SOB (shortness of breath), diaphoresis (sweating), and EKG changes. The typical patient was an upper-middle-class business executive type, member of a local country club, suffering from stresses of the competitive Manhattan business world.

Often cardiac enzymes were negative and the patient was placed on cardiac medications (nitroglycerins, beta blockers) and transferred to 5N—the floor—for a few days before discharge. Occasionally, however, someone did suffer from a massive MI, needed Swan Ganz monitoring, ECHO, and an extensive cardiac work-up with central lines placed.

My first night on call was a memorable one. All new interns had been told by the chief resident to respond to all codes—

because half of us would run in the wrong direction since none of us yet knew our way around the hospital. At 9:00 P.M., July 3, I heard the head nurse call for a code, my first resuscitation. She ran out of the room screeching, "Call a code! Call a code!" Then I saw another nurse behind the desk dial a number, whereupon the page operator notified the code team by setting off special beepers. The code team consisted of three interns on the unit, two junior residents in the unit, and one senior resident.

My out-of-condition senior resident, Jack Jacobs, ran into a room. I followed him. A man was lying on the bed without response. I heard Jack yell: "No pulse! Begin CPR!" A board was jammed under the motionless body, and chest compressions began. Jack said, "Let the new intern do it. Quick, Bea! Do you know how?" I nodded affirmatively. With that, he cupped his hands and began pushing on the man's chest about an inch above the xyphoid process.

The EKG machine was hooked up, and the monitor reading was consistent with ventricular tachycardia. "Quick! Give the man a thump!" With that, Jack punched the man in the chest. The nurses were starting lines and following Jack's instructions. A senior medical resident on call, it was his job to instruct the code.

Then, immediately, another code was called from an adjacent room. Jack ran to the other room. Beads of sweat poured from his face. His green scrubs clung to his body like a wet rag.

I noticed that I was not much better. It was my job to place the gel over the appropriate places on the patient's chest for cardiac-shocking purposes. My hands smelled like disinfectant. Blood from where I had started my first central line added color to my white jacket.

Jack dashed back to my room and yelled, "Beatrice, you stay here. I'm only in the next room. Every time the monitor makes wavy lines within this wave pattern, shock him!" I must have shocked that patient thirty times before the night was over. The odor of burning flesh filled the air. Shocking this man out of intractable VTack (ventricular tachyarrhythmia, a fatal heart rhythm) was his only chance for recovery. However, at 4:15 A.M. we pronounced him dead.

The woman that Jack worked on also died. She died at 12:15 A.M., July 4. Jack said, "For time of death write July third. Why should they [her children] always associate July Fourth with the death of their mother?"

The night moved quickly by without any discernible separation from day. I felt dirty and hungry. I grabbed a cup of cool coffee from the counter at the nurses' station. It had been left over from the night before.

"Beatrice!" I heard my name being called. "Time for morning rounds."

I grabbed my stethoscope. Making a last-ditch effort to look presentable, I put on lipstick as I ran down the hall. One minute later I caught up with my team. *Oh, no!* I thought. Rounds had already started.

Throughout all of my internship year, my mouth continued to need maintenance, checkups, prosthetic adjustments—even remodeling as the contours of my tissues changed. The long on-call nights required me to leave my prosthesis in both day and night. My tissues, given no rest from the constant rubbing of the prosthesis, became more irritated.

Again, I felt like a juggler. But now I had patients who needed help, and as I reached beyond myself to help them, I learned to cope with these new stresses that had been added to my already existing ones.

One woman I will never forget. She sat up in her bed, her blond hair draped around her shoulders, her blue eyes glistening. She appeared to be full of life, vibrant, and youthful, no more than thirty-four years of age. Those of us in charge of her knew that she suffered from a severe form of leukemia. In spite of this, she remained undaunted. Her room was filled with books, mostly ones with pictures of pretty castles decorating the English countryside. My resident and I would often chat with her. She had been an archaeologist and delighted in telling tales about her life and her explorations through foreign lands.

Simple things such as birds outside her window or live flowers in bloom made her smile. There was a magical charm about her, an appreciation of life that imbued all around her with happiness, drive, and determination.

During my long on-call nights I frequently chatted with her for a few minutes and said a few upbeat things to brighten her night. She had been requiring more frequent blood transfusions and was failing her chemotherapy. Without mentioning death, one night she asked, "What shall I do? My daughter is graduating and my immune responses are so low, I can't make it to the ceremony."

We opted for a second round of chemotherapy. This lady was a fighter. However, one night when I stopped in to see her, she looked ashen. I asked what had happened. She told me that a female patient in the same room with her had coded the night before and that she had witnessed the event. Emergency teams were unable to get her out of the room, as time did not permit.

After that, the woman was moved to a private room where the windows overlooked the lawn of the hospital grounds. But some of her joy was gone, and I sensed that her spirit was failing. One day as I was drawing her blood, she asked me if she was going to die.

I said that we all will die sometime but that we must live each day to the fullest and that all that was medically able to be done was being done. She still appeared to be sad, and I told her that I myself had faced death once and that her loneliness was natural.

She looked up at me, surprised. Every day she was surrounded by friends and family. "How did you know that I'm lonely?"

I said, "Because when a person has an inner struggle, he feels removed from the world around him."

She nodded and smiled at me. I understood. She no longer felt alone.

That week her gums bled more, and bleeding episodes increased. Then, one morning on rounds, she complained of a headache. I knew the implication and ordered a CAT scan. I calmed her fears by my own calm attitude. The scan revealed a massive bleed in the brain, and she was transferred to ICU, where she went into uncontrolled seizures and died.

After her family left the room, in private I wept over her dead body. *A woman so young, so vibrant!* I thought. It was then that I realized the fine separation that must exist between a doctor and a patient in order that the physician can continue to help the multitude. Since then, although I have genuine concern for my patients and continue to feel with and for them, I have sharpened this skill.

One afternoon, a middle-aged man with a stroke was admitted to my service. He was unable to comprehend speech or to be intelligible when he tried to speak. "Just keep him stable," my resident said. "Monitor neuro checks and leave him be."

But I thought, *He's a person too! Maybe something can be done.* So each day after work I spoke to him for a half-hour and encouraged his family to do the same. This went on for three months. A co-intern said, "That's for a speech therapist to do."

My response was, "That's for a good *doctor* to do." Patient care involves the whole person.

When he left he thanked me and told me that my help had encouraged him. Before he left North Shore, the patient was speaking simple sentences.

A young male patient with leukemia spotted me during my first week of internship. He had read articles about me. He said, "You're the doctor that got through med school despite cancer." Then he told me how his high school training had been interrupted by cancer and how he wanted to become an emergency medical technician. I encouraged him by positive reinforcement. I helped him to image himself as young, hardy, working on an ambulance. Subsequently he is in remission and is doing well.

Letters were sent to my North Shore chairman commending me for my professional expertise, my attentiveness, and my compassion, which provided my patients with medical and emotional care that gave them confidence and comfort while under treatment. These letters strengthen my strong belief in the need for the human touch in medicine. In today's society, with all of its technical advances, the need for the human touch still exists.

Before leaving the North Shore part of my internship year, I attended the fiftieth United States Presidential inauguration. A friend of mine had received two tickets, and I was invited to attend. I worked two calls in a row with a slight break in between in order to get the time off. When my plane landed in Washington, D.C., I couldn't help but be overwhelmed by the red, white, and blue decorations, the excitement that filled the air, and later, by the women dressed in fine gowns, parading through the hotel lobbies.

In the big convention halls, a national prayer service of thanksgiving was held. After that, major orchestras entertained the crowds. Suddenly all performers silenced and a marching band entered. A man's voice boomed, "Now introducing the president of the United States of America!" What a dream come true for this man—to head a whole nation!

My move to Memorial Sloan-Kettering Cancer Center came in the spring of that year. Never before had I seen such a place! The automatic doors opened into an entrance from which one took an escalator up to a spacious lobby. The lobby was decorated with flowering plants. At all hours of the day and night, peace and serenity permeated the atmosphere. Priests, ministers, rabbis, and doctors exchanged glances in the halls while patients' families paced in waiting rooms. This was the world-renowned cancer center, and I was now a part of it! With pride I placed my new ID on my white coat and took the elevator to the medical floor on which I was stationed.

One night on call, around 3:00 A.M., I entered a dark, isolated room. A patient, jaundiced from metastatic liver cancer, lay rigid on his bed. As I was only a covering physician, he was not my primary patient. A young woman with long, dark, wavy hair knelt beside him. Her hands were clenched in desperation. Upon hearing me approach, she quickly got up, straightened her skirt, and tried to clear her throat. "He's dead, isn't he?" she asked.

I listened for heart sounds, respirations, and felt for a pulse. "Yes," I said. "I'm afraid so."

Tears flooded her face. "He was so good. Why did he have to suffer so much?" Her brown eyes questioned mine.

I couldn't answer her question then, and perhaps I never will. But I gave her my listening ear, my concern, my empathy. I touched her hand and silently prayed: "Help this person cope with her loss, dear Lord. Help her to let go." Her mother and brother joined her in her sorrow shortly after that.

Months later the daughter wrote to thank me for my words of comfort, ". . . for your caring support and friendship (as well as your professionalism) will always be remembered with deep gratitude."

I folded that letter into my drawer, and today as I read it, I can't help but think, *It's one human helping another.* I might never see some of these people again, but just to touch their lives, even for a moment, gives me a sense of fulfillment. And I remember again that young intern who had sat by my bed at Yale the night before my surgery. Acts of kindness influence people and set up a chain reaction.

All people, whatever their cultures, share certain common needs. My first day on service, my resident introduced me to my patients. He pointed into one room and, indicating the patient, said, "She's unresponsive, won't be much trouble. She has a brain tumor and is admitted now for seizure control."

Later that day as I passed by her room, I heard her cry,

"Ma . . . Ma . . . Ma . . . Ma . . ." I ran to her. She clasped my hand and said, "Mama." I began to talk to her.

One of the nurses said, "She only speaks Italian." I spoke to her in my high school Italian, and I thought I saw a smile on her face. Each day after that I visited her and talked to her even though she did not reply. Then, one day, I was called to see her. She lay on her bed, contorted out of shape, seizing with tonic clonic posturing. I gave her IV doses of phenobarbital. Her seizures quieted, but she began screaming, and tears filled her eyes. I tried to comfort her with soft conversation. She seemed to quiet when I talked.

Two weeks later her daughters wheeled her by me in the nurses' station, and one of them said, "So you're the physician who speaks Italian to our mother!"

"How do you know about that?" I asked.

"She told us," was the reply.

I looked at my patient. Her seizures were controlled now and she smiled at me. "Your attempts to communicate with me were very comforting," she said.

A poignant picture flashes across my mind when I recall a lovely middle-aged woman sitting by the bedside of her comatose husband as he lay dying. Catheter, IV lines, and NG tubes invaded his body. He remained still in his bed except for occasional grunts. She seemed unaware of his unresponsive state and continued to read his mail to him. Occasionally the man opened his eyes only to close them again and drift off into his dreamworld existence.

"Why do you sit there and read to him?" I asked. I could see the terrible strain that she was under. "He is cortically dead and only responds reflexively."

Even though her husband's condition had been thoroughly explained to her, she continued to read his mail to him every day for weeks. He remained in his vegetative state.

Finally one day I was called. Her husband was no longer breathing, and I pronounced him dead at 5:00 P.M. I watched as she held his hand until the last bit of life left him. Then, with a muffled cry, she scooped his wasted body into her arms. I knew that this was the man who had held her in his arms thirty years before at a ball and had asked her to be his wife. Now, thirty years later, he lay motionless, lifeless, on his bed while she knelt beside him, weeping.

Internship was approaching an end. June drew to a close, and a new July was on the way. I received letters welcoming me into my neurology residency; it was to begin that July at New York Hospital, of which Memorial Sloan-Kettering Cancer Center was an affiliate. At last I would be immersed in my own field! I anticipated learning to care for patients with diseases of the nervous system, seizures, movement disorders, strokes, back pain, headache, and a host of other neurologic abnormalities. I was not unhappy to say good-bye to internship. It had prepared me well, but it had been a grueling experience.

A celebration at a Long Island country club was held in honor of those successfully completing medical internship. My brother accompanied me, and I received my diploma with pride. Through strength, devotion, dedication, perseverance, and imaging a goal, I had accomplished yet another dream. And dreams are like an endless staircase to paradise.

# Chapter Fourteen

IT WAS July 1, 1985, and I was about to take another step, neurology residency at New York Hospital. About fifteen neurology residents gathered in a conference room where Jerry Swift, M.D., the chairman, introduced us to one another by a brief description. He referred to my neuroanatomy research but emphasized my interest in the handicapped. "Never be late for morning report or the doors will be locked," warned the more senior residents. "Dr. Swift runs a strict department."

My life revolved around my work except for an occasional workout at a nearby gym or an evening chat with a friend. I was looking forward to the staff visit from the *Lehigh Alumni Bulletin*. They were to take pictures at New York Hospital for my article, "A Gift of Healing, Painfully Earned." They arrived, cameras in hand, and followed me throughout a typical working day. That fall, the article met with success, and letters from people who said that my enthusiasm, hope, and courage inspired them to keep going continued to crowd my mailbox. I replied to each letter personally, thinking to myself that every person has the same potential for strength. When one taps that potential, one reaps valuable rewards.

Some of the people who whote to me identified with my problem. Others were inspired by the article. Still others were moved to make copies of the article and distribute them among friends and neighbors. They hoped that it would bring "a gift of healing" or even a glimmer of hope. If that article or this book encourages even one person, then I am happy that I have written my story. It is my prayer that it will help many.

Inspired by these letters, I continued my daily life as a resident. One night I remember being paged to see a Russian diplomat with a new-onset stroke. His wife, blond and attractive, spoke only Russian and watched silently as I interviewed her husband. He stated that he felt his tongue get thick, his face grow numb, during a hot UN debate. We placed him on appropriate medications, and he did well.

After his discharge from the hospital, I drew his blood on several occasions. We frequently chatted about world events and our personal philosophies. Even though we argued, I grew to like his spunk. To recuperate, he visited Moscow. Several months later, as I stood in the hall of the hospital, I saw a man in a big black fur coat approach me. It was my Russian patient. He was carrying a small gift-wrapped package. "This is for you," he said. "Merry Christmas!"

I opened the present later that night in my Manhattan studio, part of the hospital housing. How nice, I thought, a perfume bottle with a pretty label, lettered all in Russian. I opened the bottle and smelled. Not much scent. Oh, well! The women in Russia probably have less than we, more simple tastes, I thought, as I splashed the perfume over my body.

The next day I showed the attending-in-charge my nice gift, and he laughed. "Beatrice, that's vodka!" I blushed and headed for clinic.

I always enjoyed working with clinic patients. One man in

particular at New York Hospital had a very difficult seizure disorder to control. Multiple medications failed, and he spent much of his time half drugged from the sedative effects of phenobarbital.

"Dr. Engstrand," he said, "I want to work, but I can't. I don't feel like a person anymore. There's no meaning in my life."

"Oh, yes there is," I reprimanded him. "Look to the positives. You have a friend who loves you, and you *are* capable of doing volunteer work."

"You think so? Who would recommend me?"

"I will."

The man smiled, but at the same time, a tear formed, and he tried to conceal it. After that, during his clinic visits, we chatted about his new work, and I could tell by his manner that his life had taken on new meaning.

Across the street from New York Hospital is Memorial Sloan-Kettering. As part of my neurology training, I was to rotate there, where I had worked before as a medical intern. Now I would return as a neurology resident.

Memorial has a pain service under the division of neurology. The service consults on patients in severe pain from all types of cancer. Routinely these patients are managed from outpatient clinics where the physicians-in-charge manipulate oral doses of narcotics, including such potent drugs as morphine and Levo-Dromoran. Most patients respond to such therapy. Those who don't respond are admitted to the hospital. Several alternative therapies can be tried in the hospital, such as the administration of IV narcotics or the performance of certain procedures. One of these procedures is known as a cordotomy, in which nerves that carry pain to the brain are severed. Cordotomies are not always successful, although they do have a relatively high rate of success at Memorial.

One night on call, an elective admission arrived for pain control. She was a thirty-two-year-old woman who had undergone bilateral mastectomies seven years before.

Upon entering her room, I found the shades pulled for the

evening and heard sniffles, little tiny sobs, high-pitched as
though from a baby bird. A body, alone, lay face-down on the
bed, not moving, but breathing. This patient had been lying on
her stomach for two years, unable to turn over because she had
no supporting structures left to her back. Cancer had eroded
her entire lower spine and pelvis.

My third-year student accompanied me into the room. She
was on a four-week rotation through neurology, and everything was new to her. Before entering the room, I had decided
that the student should follow this patient in order to learn how
to manage those in intractable pain.

As we moved closer to the patient's bed, my medical student
mumbled to me, "What's that terrible stench?" Pus and blood
were running down the side of the patient's bed.

In spite of her agonizing pain, the patient happily informed
me that now, at Memorial, she was going to have a procedure
done, a cordotomy, and would no longer suffer from pain. She
had already failed IV drips and was a very unusual patient in
the fact that she was in the end stage of a decayed body with a
completely intact mind. I found out later from the pain service
that she had requested that the drugs not dull her mind if at all
possible, because she enjoyed conversations with her mother.

But now she had a fever, and after consultation all the doctors agreed that the oozing from her leg indicated a bad infection, and that she could not be a candidate for the cordotomy.
Further tests were done, and we discovered a possible abscess
cavity tracking from her upper right thigh to her abdominal
cavity. Cancer had eaten away enough of the bone for the pus
to track through.

We concurred that if we could drain the abscess, she could be
a candidate for the cordotomy. The surgeons feared that she
would be left with a gaping wound that would not heal. But the
patient wanted the cordotomy, and the only way she could
have it was for us to clear her infection and rid her of the
abscess. The attending told me to pursue an aggressive work-
up on the patient.

She went into surgery to have the abscess drained. Down in the operating room, however, as soon as the surgeons cut her skin, she started to bleed out, with blood going out of her as fast as a sink faucet in full force. Surgery was now impossible.

When she arrived back on the floor, it was my job to pump blood into her as fast as it poured out in order to keep her alive. She had no IV access, but a surgeon started a central line, and blood products poured in. Tumor eroded her bladder, and massive blood clots in her urine required her to have chronic bladder irrigation.

A meeting was held to determine her code status, and the attending declared her unable to be coded because she couldn't be turned over and resuscitated. When I left Memorial to go to the Hospital of Special Surgery (HSS), that patient was still being maintained on IV pain medications.

In a nearby room a patient remained in isolation. Caution signs covered the entrance; an AIDS patient resided there. I had to draw his blood, and we began to talk. I said, "You must be lonely in here."

"Boy!" he said. "If you only knew!" His cachectic body, gaunt facial features, and blond hair depicted a skeleton if ever I saw one. "You know, my lover doesn't even talk to me. My family has disowned me, and society shuns me. I wish I were dead. I'm in a living hell. Isolated from people by gloves, masks, gowns, I'm ostracized by all." He pleaded with me. "I'm a human being in this body. I have feelings."

I held his hand and looked into his eyes. Strange, I thought, when I began med school, AIDS as we know it did not exist. It's a relatively new and fatal disease. Seldom in the history of medicine does a disease confront society with such magnitude and depth, eliciting fear and dread from all sectors. This man was right. Only understanding and research will help him.

For the most part I function normally, but I live each day with a hidden problem that does make me feel vulnerable. While on call another night, I was paged to the bed-holding area of Memorial—it's like their emergency room. I was examining a patient when suddenly I heard a snap, and my prosthesis fell down in my mouth. Embarrassed, I grasped it. My supporting clamp had broken. Just when I begin to think of myself as a completely normal person, reality surfaces and reminds me of my handicap. But I refuse to give in. That night I ran home and grabbed my spare prosthesis, which fit tight but was uncomfortable in my mouth, and scheduled an emergency visit with Dr. Stein the next day.

After that visit, reminded once again of my limitations, I wanted to do something pleasurable. I went to Peppermint Park, a nearby ice cream parlor on the east side of Manhattan. There, I would just relax and relish a fattening treat.

I entered the parlor and sat at a small table. The waiter asked for my order. To his surprise, I said, "Give me the most fattening thing on the menu."

A few minutes later, he arrived with a big piece of chocolate cake, whipped cream, and scoops of ice cream. Delighted, I eagerly began to devour the mounds of calories. Meanwhile, a young man and his little girl sat next to my table. His little girl chuckled when she saw an adult eating all that ice cream. The man looked up, and we began to talk.

He was a pleasant man, casually dressed, well versed. He told me that he was a businessman, and I told him that I was a resident at Memorial Sloan-Kettering Cancer Center. In the course of that conversation I discussed the plight of the AIDS patients. The man listened intently as I promoted humanism in medicine. "You know, you should write an article about that," he said.

I replied that I already had written an article, and referred to my Lehigh article that fall.

"Great!" he exclaimed. "If you wouldn't mind, deliver it at my condo. Leave it with the doorman, and if I like it, I'll let my agent see it." This man was influential not only in the business world but in the literary and theatrical worlds as well. A phone message the next day brought tears to my eyes. "Beatrice!

Loved the article. Gave it to my agent to review." The rest is now history; this book is based on that article.

In the interim, my first year of neurology was approaching an end. New York Hospital held a special place in my heart, yet my life was taking a different direction. I was going to leave New York Hospital and transfer to Brooklyn's Downstate Medical Center–Kings County Hospital (now the State University of New York Science Center at Brooklyn), where I would complete the last two years of my training. I had already interviewed for a position there, and the atmosphere and the particular problems that I would be facing were different from those I had known before. But I felt that this would add another enriching dimension to my life.

Dr. Arthur Caliandro, minister of Marble Collegiate Church, which I attend when I am in Manhattan, encouraged me to nurture the part of me that was *me* and not to lose track of where I was going. He and I talked often together, and we have become close friends, sharing a common belief in positive thinking, imaging, enthusiasm, and joy in life itself.

Father Richard Devine of St. John's University also helped me to keep my thoughts centered upon my major goal: to be as fine a clinician as I possibly can be and to delight in sharing my life with others. In spite of all of my efforts to keep cheerful, there were times when I felt severely depressed. And it was during those times that I knew that I could always turn to Father Devine for help. He had befriended my brother during his undergraduate and law school years, and now he has become my friend, too. When he is not at the university teaching theology, Father Devine is a regular volunteer at an AIDS center in the inner city. Often we have friendly discussions about ethics in medicine, and I value his opinion. Therefore, it was a blessing for me to be able to speak freely with him about the new turn that my medical career was taking.

However, saying good-bye to New York Hospital was not easy. My last full day there I spent at the Hospital of Special

Surgery. One can see the East River flowing in the distance, because the hospital abuts it. HSS is a hospital that specializes in orthopedic and related problems. At 7:30 A.M. I had a meeting with Gary Schriver, M.D., my attending. He greeted me warmly, chatted over coffee, and then we went off to clinic.

After clinic I went to Dr. Swift's office. "Dr. Swift," I said, "I want to thank you for the experience I have had here, and I now look forward to moving on."

"Make sure you chart your life well and develop your own potentials, Beatrice. You have many talents," he said, adding that he had enjoyed having me there and urging me to keep in touch.

I then walked over to Memorial Sloan-Kettering Cancer Center to say good-bye to Dr. Gold. I entered the halls of MSKCC in a new light. This was the lobby of the hospital I knew well. To this center for cancer and allied diseases many people come, in their last plea for life, their last chance, their last hope. As I walked through the lobby, I sensed the hospital's original mission. It had been built as a refuge, as a center for hope with an emphasis on the humanitarian needs of the ill and the dying.

Heading to Dr. Gold's office, I took the elevator to the seventh floor. To my right, I smell familiar smells—of cleaning fluids, of the odor that that floor takes on—familiar smells but not unpleasant. But I didn't make my right onto the ward where I had worked at the nurses' station with the resident and where I had slept when I was a visiting medical student. I turned instead to the left and entered the doors beyond which the clinicians have their offices. I walked about two thirds of a block and came to Dr. Gold's office on my left. But the door to his office was shut, and a secretary greeted me. "What do you want?"

"It's my last day here. I'd like to say good-bye to Dr. Gold."

Her eyes swept over me for a brief moment before she knocked on his door. I walked in, and seeing me, he got up from his desk and we shook hands. "Good-bye," I said. "Thank you for everything."

"Keep in touch," he said.

After that, before leaving for my apartment, I called Dr. Shriver. We had a cup of coffee and a final chat. I would miss working with him.

Walking back to my apartment for the last time, I wondered what new challenges lay ahead for me at Kings County Hospital.

# Chapter Fifteen

LESS THAN A year after the publication of the Lehigh article, I entered Downstate Medical Center–Kings County Hospital for my second year of neurology residency. At kings County Hospital, most of my work is done for the poor and the underprivileged.

In many ways, this has been my most rewarding work of all. A word of encouragement, a bit of cutting through the red tape, humanism tempering the awesome impersonal powers of technology—these, too, are gifts of healing.

I had been warned that working at Kings County Hospital would be a culture shock, but I soon felt at home in my new locale. Hundreds of thousands of homeless and uninsured people go there every year seeking medical care that they so desperately need.

Even though I had the advantages of a middle-class family, the concept of poverty was no stranger to me. My mother, while I was young, taught me to appreciate people of all backgrounds. "People who are poor have sometimes missed out on opportunities," she would say.

Kings County Hospital exposed me to America's poor. As a municipal hospital, it fills a great need. Through my work there I sensed that I was becoming involved in something special.

My role became clear through my encounters with patients. Poor people, with the same feelings as others, feel limits to their dreams. *Why should that be?* I asked myself. They, too, should have an opportunity for unlimited horizons. They, too, should receive encouragement in their endeavors and have active role models. To truly help them, one must be aware of their needs.

The doctors servicing them, my new friends, consist of a hardworking, down-to-earth, sincere, family-oriented group. Their warmth extends into the workplace. All of us come from varied backgrounds, yet we all work together for a common goal. This first year at Kings County Hospital was to be my first exposure to battlefield neurology.

The emergency room rotation seems to capture the pulse of the inner city. The emergency room (ER) consists of many rooms. There are rooms for just men, others just for women. There are cast and X-ray rooms, and an asthma room. A treatment room serves minor trauma—lacerations, minor bruises and bangs. Then there is C1. C1 is the ICU (intensive care unit) section of the emergency room; it consists of both surgical and medical. People with major trauma and severe injuries are rushed to the surgical side by emergency services. On occasion, people from motor vehicle accidents come in with severed arms or legs. One can hear the screams and groans of victims of shoot-outs, stabbings, and gang fights. Across the hall, on the medical side, are patients with status epilepticus (uncontrolled seizures), congestive heart failure, signs of herniation (brain swelling), and a variety of other disorders.

One day, while carrying the ER beeper, I said to myself, *All is quiet. I might as well study.* What a mistake! As soon as I became engrossed in my reading, the beeper sounded. "Dr. Engstrand, we have a consult for you." The voice on the other end hesitated, then continued. "Not just one, but a whole truckload of prisoners. They've gotten in a major motor vehicle accident. Come quick!"

When I arrived, every room in the ER was filled, and police were all over. One couldn't even budge. Two incidents had occurred simultaneously. In addition to the truck accident, two policemen had been involved in a shoot-out. Within minutes all had converged on Kings County Hospital ER. Many of these patients required definitive lifesaving care. With all of this trauma, neurology was one of the services most needed. Head trauma, altered consciousness, muscle and nerve injuries, necessitated my help. Immediately I swung into action and set to work with trauma teams and neurosurgery.

Television cameras, reporters, and Mayor Koch were there. There was blood all over, and I saw a body being wheeled out. Police and prisoners were lying next to one another on stretchers. I thought, *What a weird commentary on human nature! They're fighting opposite causes, and when they face death, if there's a major crisis, their bodies lie beside one another.*

In the midst of all this commotion, I heard a voice call, "Bea! Bea!" Looking up from a prisoner I was examining, I saw the familiar figure of one of my peers. "Can I help you?" he asked. "I heard it's really busy down here."

"I can manage," I said. I knew he was on a busy service, and it was very nice of him to have offered. No one had sent him. He had come down on his own.

The prisoner I was examining whined, "Doc, my back hurts. I can't walk." I elicited a painful stimulus from him. He withdrew appropriately and then tried to kick me. He had been feigning weakness, hoping that he wouldn't get to the courtroom on time for the trial he was involved with and that a mistrial would be declared. But I cleared him medically and he glowered at me, his face livid with rage.

When I got home to my apartment building that night, I was confronted with, "How come you saved those prisoners?" "You should let them die. Work slowly. How would people know?"

I said, "If I did something like that, I'd lose my license."

"You don't have to tell people."

I shook my head. "It's not my job to judge them," I said.

When I was in medical school, I had been instructed not to make personal judgments—to let the courts decide who was innocent and who was guilty. At that time, I had wondered why my professors addressed that issue. Now I knew why when I heard this angered person muttering, "They're just going to go out and shoot others."

In the quiet of my studio apartment, which overlooked the hospital, I read a letter that I had just received from my former attending at the Hospital of Special Surgery:

> Just a quick note of thanks—and a wish for smooth sailing in your new locale.
>
> We can't be everything to everyone—time and individual capabilities simply don't allow. You have wonderful enthusiasm, interest, and fearless questioning that will always make you a terrific physician. I'm glad to be a member of the same profession . . .

As I folded his letter into my top dresser drawer, I thought about the orderly, almost patrician surroundings of the New York Hospital complex, a sharp contrast to the violence and horror that I had witnessed earlier that day.

A slight feeling of nostalgia swept over me, but I knew one thing for certain. Here, at Kings County Hospital, I was learning to be the best doctor that I could possibly be. I was seeing an endless number of patients with very real problems, many of which were compounded by poverty. In addition to treating strokes, comas, and a host of neurological disorders, I was treating the victims of gunshot wounds, stabbings, street violence. The experience that I was gaining and the training that I was receiving here gave me an incredible sense of confidence in my medical skills. I believed in myself, in my abilities as a physician. And that's a wonderful feeling. Each day, I promised myself, I would picture the good around me and help others to do the same.

I work closely with a transplant team. I know that one of the team members himself is alive today because of a successful kidney transplant received years earlier. "You can give life to others," I hear the transplant team say to parents of a brain-dead boy who has suffered a fatal gunshot wound to the head. "Kidneys, heart, eyes, liver, will save someone else. Your son is young but there is no hope. He's dead."

The brain dead note requires a neurologist to perform an apnea test. That test meets certain criteria that determine if any brain activity is left. If not, a person is declared brain dead, with no hope for survival.

The boy lay still. He was unable to breathe on his own, his head was bandaged from surgical attempts to save his life, yet his heart continued to beat.

Many die needlessly from the shortage of vital, usable organs that remain in a body whose brain is dead and which fulfills the death criteria. After the brain dies, other vital and transplant-able organs remain alive for a period of time. It is then that a dead patient's organs can be taken—giving the gift of life to another. The body is given full respect, and the organs are harvested by simple, nonmutilating surgical procedures. It is a touching and wonderful memorial.

My work as a physician can sometimes be fraught with frustrations, but I try to maintain a sense of humor. One day while on ward rounds, the attending and several residents approached a small woman in a wheelchair. She looked at all of us. When the attending went to examine her, she said, "Oh my God, you beat me up yesterday. You came and stuck me. No more! No, sir! No! That's enough. No sirree!" she said, and we could not do much of an exam on her. That was apparently her impression of a neurologist. I found the situation rather humorous.

Humor, enthusiasm, goodwill, and a listening ear have helped some of my clinic patients immensely. My very first clinic patient at Kings County Hospital arrived at my office early in July. Tall, thin, skittish, he became skeptical when seeing a new doctor. I assured him that I was there to help. He came to the neurology clinic for a seizure disorder and needed his medications adjusted. I spoke to him about his home situation and learned that this patient was being denied disability insurance. He was too ill to work and was not malingering. I told him not to worry, that I would fill out necessary papers and phone respective agencies as needed. Relieved, the man gave me a hardy handshake as he left the office. The months that followed proved trying for both of us. I defended his character, provided agencies with necessary information, and thought, *Here's a man who really needs help. What bureaucracy!*

Finally, hard work paid off. One day a clinic nurse reported that this man had arrived at the clinic. I thought, *How strange! He's not scheduled for today.* But I agreed to see him.

"Call for him now," I said to the nurse. As I looked up from my desk, I saw him, his face beaming with joy. He carried a pot of yellow tulips and a thank you card, which he proudly presented to me. He had received his disability check. I knew he could ill afford the gift he had given to me. Touched, I told him I would always treasure it. The tulips are alive and grow in my yard today.

The ill need medical help, but their practical concerns must also be addressed. One day a social worker stopped me in the hall. "Hey! Remember that patient you saw the other day in the ER?"

I said, "Which one?"

He said, "The one who was retarded. She came with her mother, who was also vaguely retarded."

"Oh, yeah!" I said.

I had been called to see a cerebral palsy patient in her late thirties. The patient, in a wheelchair, was having poorly controlled seizures. The mother complained, "I can't manage her at home without assistance." She stared at me, waiting for my reply.

"Why can't you get help?" I questioned.

She said, "Because nobody's there to give it to me."

I said, "Well, I'll try to help you out." I knew that it is very important to insure that the home environment is as conducive as possible to the care that people need.

I called Social Work, and social services showed up. I told them, "These people need help. Try to see what we can get. I'll do anything you need. Just give me the forms." Right there, I filled out all the forms, saying that the daughter needed assistance with the activities of daily living. Social Work then submitted the forms.

Now, three days later, this social worker, meeting me in the hall, said, "Well, you did a good deed."

I said, "What do you mean?"

He said, "That family finally got the care that they needed. Someone will go to the house, help clean, and feed and assist the daughter with her daily living. Now the patient won't have to be institutionalized."

That was a very unusual case. In general, applicants for disability and aid wait weeks, months, and sometimes longer. That is, if they get any assistance at all. Disability funding is difficult to get. There is a lot of red tape, and many forms to be filled out. One must buck the system.

Frequently I give my work number to deserving patients and encourage them to have the agencies call me so that I can substantiate their medical needs and get them help as quickly as possible.

At times, it is difficult to place people in day-care or rehabilitation centers. More places are needed to help the handicapped person acclimate to society. Brilliant minds, enthusiastic spirits, future contributors to society, are not being given a chance. One patient, a twenty-year-old with cerebral palsy, beamed, "Doc, I just graduated." He had just completed a special school. "Now I'm going to go to a center and receive training for a skilled job." A few months later the center phoned to tell

me that they had refused him because he had difficulty con-
trolling his urine.

I said, "He's had that handicap all his life. He wears diapers
and manages well. He never makes a mess."

The voice on the other end remained adamant.

And I said, "What do you do with people who wear colos-
tomies?" The person on the other end did not reply.

Needless to say, the patient returned to my office crushed.
"Don't worry," I told him. "We will find a way."

Another follow-up that day was a young girl, about fourteen,
who had been sent over to the ER to be organically cleared for
her headaches. From her history and medical exam, I suspected
meningitis. When I admitted her to neurology to have a spinal
tap done, she became frightened, and I held her hand and
talked to her. I told her that she was young, that she still had
a chance for a good life. I told her that I had confidence in her
and that I had faith in her and that I was a friend who would
stand by her. She sensed my sincerity and appreciated that
little gleam of hope that I had given to her.

She did have meningitis. After treatment, she was referred
back to the psychiatric building for detoxification of her drug
disorder and for guidance. On her way back to the Psychiatric
Institute, she came and gave me a big hug and a kiss and said
that I'd saved her life.

Arriving slightly late to the pediatric neurology clinic, I found
a patient waiting in my room. He had Romberg syndrome, a
hemifacial atrophy, a wasting of the facial muscle. Romberg
syndrome can be associated with seizures, slow development,
headache, and a receding hairline. Previous tests had confirmed this disorder. I treated his organic problem and scheduled him for an EEG, which would indicate whether or not he
had seizures. But most important here was that this child had
a facial abnormality. He was only thirteen years old; the hair
had receded from his forehead, and his face was very asym-
metric.

After asking the patient to leave the room, I discussed the

case with the mother. The kids in the school poked fun at him, she told me. She said that he had been a brilliant honor student and that he was starting to misbehave in school because he thought nobody cared about him. In short, he was giving up. Sensitive to her concerns, I told her that something had happened to my face (I didn't tell her what) and that I had been traumatized in the first year of medical school, that people had thought, at first, that I had been hit by a Mack truck. I expressed how devastating it had been to me. I told her how I had had to relearn that *I am who I am* regardless of what my face looks like, and that regardless of how I feel, I can still make a presentation to the world. "If all the handicapped people quit, I wouldn't be here to help you today," I said. "Do you want me to share this with your son?"

"Yes. Oh, will you please talk to him," she implored, "because the kids at school taunt him and say, 'You'll never get anywhere. You'll never go to college because your face is so funny.' " And she went on, "When he hears from you, and you're a doctor, it will mean a lot to him."

So I called him in. "Listen," I said, "I don't usually tell people this, but I want to tell *you* this. When I was younger, I had trouble with *my* face. You take a good look at it." And I took my glasses off. I said, "You see how swollen this side is?" as I pointed to my left side. "And how much wider this eye is? I even have to wear an appliance that helps me to talk. Without it, I can't even talk. It happens that I had some trauma in the first year of medical school, and it affected my looks and the way I felt about myself. And I didn't go out on dates or think of myself as pretty or normal, pretty much the way that you feel." He nodded. I continued, "One day I realized that I am the person who's inside of me. The glow from within me comes out on my face, and *people will see only what I see about myself.* So, if you accept yourself, other people will accept you too. However, you are a child, and kids make fun of people who are different. Dare to be different! Get to know yourself. Like yourself. Give of yourself. And demand the best of yourself."

I thought about my own grammar school days. I had been absent so much of the time, unable to participate in sports when I did attend, and a sudden spurt of growth had lifted me, head and shoulders, above the rest of the girls and most of the boys. Most of the time the children chose to ignore me—almost as though I didn't exist—excluding me from their conversations and their play.

It was tempting, at first, to want to pattern myself in the same mold as the other children in order that I wouldn't be singled out for ridicule. And then I realized that this would be impossible. I couldn't change my height. I couldn't change the fact that I was ill and absent.

Years later Mom told me that when the children had gathered around her to thank her for her holiday performance, one or two of them had asked how I was doing. She told them that I was in the hospital with asthma, that she hoped that I would be coming home soon, and that she knew that I would be happy to hear from any of them during the holiday vacation. As she started to leave the room, she overheard some of them talking about me.

"Why didn't she die?" one girl said.

"Why don't they just throw her into a garbage pail?"

"Throw her in the street."

Mom fled to the school nurse's office to hide her tears. And that night, when she told Dad about it, she insisted that I transfer from that school into Our Redeemer Lutheran School in Seaford at the end of the semester. Dad agreed.

At Our Redeemer Lutheran School, one teacher, Bob Brocker, taught most of the subjects for the sixth grade. He was a strict, very gifted, kindly person who really enjoyed his work, and all of the students loved him. Each morning we began the day with religious services.

Toward the end of the school year, Mom questioned Mr. Brocker, "Why is it that Bea has had such a positive experience in your class and such a dreadful experience in the other school?"

Mr. Brocker responded immediately. "Proper training and guidance from an adult. Before the end of the last semester, when I knew that Beatrice would be coming to us, I prepared the class to receive her."

"How did you do that?" Mom asked.

"Simple." Mr. Brocker smiled at her. "This may be a church school, but we don't have any angels here. We have a mix of children, some from church backgrounds, some not. A variety of races, too. And we also have love and we have discipline. My students know that I mean what I say. So I just gathered them all together one day and said, 'Listen, you guys and gals, a new student is going to join us right after Christmas. She's kind of special because she has been very sick. And she's still not strong. I want you to make her welcome and I want you to accept her immediately. If anyone here makes her uncomfortable or gives her a hard time, they will have to answer to me.' "

That semester at Our Redeemer proved to be my happiest and most rewarding school experience.

And that was when *I* learned one of the most important lessons of my life: DARE TO BE DIFFERENT! Get to know yourself. Like yourself. Give of yourself. And demand the best of yourself.

And then I thought after surgery, I had to get to know myself. I literally had to find myself, and that had been hard to do. We tend to identify ourselves with fixed images of our physical selves. And without our being aware of it, we let those images take control of our lives. Well, I had to search very deep until I found the real me. And it took a long time before I could say to myself with any conviction, "You're still there, girl. Not a shattered vestige of yourself but the whole, complete you." I had to do it in stages, because the physical deformity and the constant pain kept screaming, *We are the reality. We are the reality.*

Now I heard myself saying to my young patient, "You have to keep on going. Ignore the laughter of the other kids, as hard as it is. Handicapped people, yourself, myself, mustn't give up. If I had given up, I wouldn't be here to help you today. Now I'm a doctor. You, too, have to keep on going to help yourself as well as other handicapped people. You're intelligent, an honor student. The world needs intelligent leaders. You must go ahead." Gratefully, he held my hand. We understood each other. After that, he agreed to seek counseling.

# Chapter Sixteen

CLINIC ENDED that day and I picked up the on-call beeper. Grabbing a cup of coffee and a handful of popcorn, I went to the ER. I had been asked to see a fifteen-year-old accompanied by his father. He had been playing basketball the day before I saw him, had been hit in the chest by somebody's elbow. The next day, in the evening, he had complained of shortness of breath. Chest tightness followed, and he also had abnormal, dystonic movements. It looked like the reaction one can get from certain drugs, although he denied drug abuse. He appeared to come from a good, upstanding family, but all the books supported that he had idiosyncratic dyskinesias (abnormal movements), which responded well to the drugs that I gave him.

I told the emergency room resident to do an EKG. He wondered why a fifteen-year-old would need an electrocardiogram. I said, "Do it." Well, the EKG was abnormal, with multiple abnormal cardiac rhythms, which was consistent with, among other things, drug ingestion. The teenager was scared to death.

He finally admitted that this was his first time messing with drugs. But when he had first come in, he had denied drug ingestion.

It's particularly sad that people in the ghetto start drugs at a young age. They are born into an environment without much chance, without any financial security. It's an uphill battle for them to break through today's social barriers. They need to receive positive reinforcement for the good that they accomplish.

"I want to kill myself. That's the only answer," another young clinic patient wailed. She sat at the edge of her chair. "Pushers shove drugs. Some of my friends are crack addicts. Mom won't even let me out of the house anymore. She doesn't understand. I'm so alone. Now look!" She handed me a notice that terminated her employment.

She muttered, "Now I don't even have a job."

The sentence *I want to kill myself* kept repeating.

I thought of the street scene that she had just left, with its pimps, pushers, and prostitutes. Crime ALL OVER. Earlier that day, I had a seen a sixteen-year-old after his first time "shooting up." I reprimanded him, "IV drugs are dangerous. You can get AIDS." I was trying to scare him away from drugs because his peers were saying, "Drugs are okay."

Now I found myself admonishing the suicidal girl, "If you do kill yourself, there's no coming back. Your Mom would be devastated." But in her anguish, she couldn't reason. My efforts futile, I said firmly, "You must see a psychiatrist."

"I won't."

"You must."

"I'm not hurting anyone."

"But you're a threat to yourself."

By this time, security arrived to escort her to the psychiatry division, the G Building. The patient glared at me. She subsequently received the help that she needed.

These patients are so young. Their whole lives get messed up at such an early age. I hope that by talking to each one, by viewing them as individuals, by giving them insight into their problems, maybe at some point I can reach out and help one person, one out of twenty. Even one life changed and touched in some manner would make a difference.

Another time, a middle-aged patient arrived at the hospital with her adolescent daughter. The patient had new onset seizures. A head scan disclosed a brain tumor. A biopsy report confirmed—glioblastoma multiforme, a rapidly progressing primary nervous system cancer. Social Services, upon finding that the daughter lived alone at home with her mother, became involved with the case, and I gave a little extra.

I called the young girl into my office one day. This girl had not complained. Yet I knew that watching one's mother die could not be easy. I reflected back on Beth. It had taken me years of soul-searching to piece together the subtle warning signs. But they were there. At the time that they occurred, they seemed to be problems that were being handled, being coped with, or about to be solved. But obviously that wasn't enough. The seeds of despair were planted deep.

"Tell me about yourself," I said, looking at the young girl. Young, thin, intelligent, she was an honors student.

"I'm finding it harder to study now. Mom sleeps all the time, and when she doesn't, she yells. She's not the same person anymore. We live together. Just the two of us. Sometimes my brother visits. Last night Mom stood on the top of the stairs and threw darts at us."

In addition to distant relatives and friends, this young girl often turned to me for advice during those trying months. Finally one day I received a call.

"It's my mom! She's dying."

I arrived at the room. With her craniotomy scar visible, the patient lay stretched flat on the bed, her belly distended. My internal medicine friends informed me of their diagnosis: "Perforated abdomen. An acute surgical emergency." Her pressure was now dropping, and emergency measures were withheld. Weeks after the patient died, I continued to hear from the

daughter. With constant encouragement, she plugged away
with her studies and is now doing well.

Frequently at Kings County Hospital, we are called to consult
on patients with AIDS. A twenty-three-year-old man had been
diagnosed as having AIDS in January 1986, when he first was
discovered to have pneumocystic pneumonia. A CAT scan of
his head showed a toxoplasmosis lesion for which he received
multiple medications. According to one of my peers who knew
this patient, nothing had changed in his exam. Yet he had come
to the emergency room this night, and I wondered why. I
thought for a second and said, "You're bothered by something." I had broken the ice because I was very friendly.

When he spoke, his voice was tinged with sadness. "The
nurse didn't even want to touch me. She was skittish. She
moved away."

I said, "Don't take it personally. She's been working a double
shift."

And he said, "Yes." And he looked at me with his sunken
eyes and said, "I feel terrible."

I said, "Why?"

And he said, "My child is eighteen months old. I have an
eighteen-month-old son and he has AIDS-related complex.
He's gonna die, and it's all my fault." Tears came to his eyes.

I said, "Well, no living being is fully guilty. You have re-
morse. You repent. Beyond that, you can't tear yourself up. No
one deserves to do that." We discussed the fact that through
research, one day a breakthrough might be achieved. "You're
still a living human being with good points," I told him.

He was encouraged. I gave him a handshake and let him
know that I understood how he felt. The fact that I had just lent
a listening ear to his loneliness, that I understood the suffering,
the internal turmoil that AIDS patients face, made him feel
better. In addition, I came up with some good physical therapy
suggestions and range-of-motion exercises. Then I wrote a prescription for him to get a walker for his persistent weakness.

He implored, "Will you pray for me?"

I hadn't told him that I was religious, but I did agree that I would pray for him. He felt much relieved.

AIDS victims seek help each day from Kings County. Often neurology consults on them or diagnoses them for the first time. A person is at risk if he or she is an IV drug abuser, a homosexual, or the recipient of multiple blood transfusions. The list of risk factors continues to grow. Neurological manifestations of AIDS include, among other things, a thought disorder, new onset of seizures, encephalitis, meningitis, and primary cancers of the nervous system. Health care workers are advised to exercise special cautions with their blood products, to double-glove, and to wear a gown and mask.

Young people are dying each day by this fatal disease. It can run either a rapid or a slow course. I remember a patient who had died two weeks after filming a TV commercial. I also know people alive after several years with this disease.

When faced with the diagnosis, people often deny it. Special antifungal and antibiotic agents are now available which help to slow the course of this immunocompromising disease. However, as it continues to wipe away the immune system, the patient is unable to mount responses to fight off even simple infections. Frequently the patient suffers from pneumonia and from oral candidiasis, a white fungus in the mouth which can make eating painful. Not only do their bodies fail them, but also their social support structure crumbles. Alone in their rooms, isolated from friends, stigmatized, too ill to take care of their wants, they waste away. Often many victims watch their few remaining friends die. They know that their destiny will soon follow a similar course.

A need exists for a concerned public to help these people and to try to prevent the further spread of this fatal virus by any known preventative measures.

The resident whom I was supervising that night called from Downstate Medical Center to ask that I assist her in the discussion she was having with a patient's family about whether or not to resuscitate their young daughter, who was fatally afflicted by multisystem disease. In the care of a patient, communication is very important, so that teamwork can occur each step of the way. I answered all the parents' questions and explained that their daughter had no cortical or brainstem function left. "No matter what happens, all you will have left is a heart pumping in a body," I said. "Do you really want to prolong this agony any longer?"

The father asked, "What will be gained from resuscitation?"

I said, "Nothing in her case. If she lived, it would just be a matter of time." It was agreed that this patient was not to be resuscitated.

Riker's Island inmates frequently seek admission to Kings County Hospital through the emergency room, because they know that once admitted, they will be away from the prison for a time.

The prison wards of Kings County Hospital are secured. In order to enter, one must pass tight security. A guard stands watch at a desk in an alcove. He scans anyone seeking to enter. Upon entering, one passes through a series of cagelike doors, shows proper ID, and after passing inspection, is permitted entry. The prisoners—drug pushers, pimps, and the like—are in open wards of about ten men. They are free to wander around the rooms in hospital pajamas. Security guards are all over. Cigarettes and little TVs are available. On occasion, I am called to consult.

In the midhours of a night on call, I was summoned to do a consult on a twenty-one-year-old man, handcuffed legs and hands, who had been attacked by six other inmates and beaten up at Riker's Island. He was in a small room, usually used for blood drawing. Four policemen stood nearby with guns. Another inmate, lying on a bench, waited to be seen by a different specialist. *Normal exam*, I wrote. *No further diagnostic work needed*. But the prisoner begged to stay for the night.

I said, "I can't do that. The hospital is no place to escape from your problems." I walked away, the policeman accompanying me, and I said, "What a sad thing."

The policeman nodded. "He's worried about being beaten up again."

By this time I had left the prisoner, and patients were spilling into the waiting area of the emergency room. Many of them slept on benches or sat on the floor. Mothers with toddlers, and babies in carriages, also waited. There are too few M.D.s for so many patients.

Many times I see diseases exacerbated as a result of poverty, lack of education, ignorance, and self-neglect. In the emergency room I frequently work side by side with my medical resident peers. We see diabetics in coma or hypertensives with major intracranial hemorrhages that might have been averted had medical advice been followed properly. Many fail to give their bodies proper attention until the situation becomes acute.

One resident told me about a comatose patient he had seen the year before. The young man and his family waited outside the doors of the intensive care unit. The neurology resident and the neurosurgery resident were trying to tell the family that the man was in a deep stage of coma. The family, much poorer than the average Kings County poor, and illiterate as well, said, "Yes, Doc. But when will he be able to eat again?"

Some of these patients speak Spanish, Creole, and island dialects. My first patient from the West Indies, during my first months at Kings County Hospital, had been a man with severe prostatic cancer that had metastasized to his spine, and he suffered from cord compression. Radiation scars had darkened areas of the skin where he had already received radiation therapy. His thirty-year-old daughter and her stepmother were concerned about how he was doing. The daughter, sobbing in hysteria, told me in private, "He can't die! He's my father!"

I admitted the patient to the hospital under the medicine service. There, he was to receive oncology consultation and management of his multiple medical problems.

Months later in the emergency room, I was called to see him again. I knew he had been receiving maximal medical and surgical treatment. The son told me that the father wished to go

back to the West Indies to die. He asked if he was stable enough
to make the trip. I said, "Yes, he is." The father had told me
that he was holding on for his daughter but that he wanted to
die. I told the daughter to let her father go in peace and not to
make the father feel guilty about dying. I encouraged her to
exercise that special self-discipline that enables one to say, "I
care for you enough to set you free." The son was very happy
about that.

The plan was to have the doctors in the Indies contact me if
necessary. Tears came to the father's eyes, and he grabbed my
hand and said, "Thank you very much." I got psychiatric care to
help the daughter better deal with her father's impending death.

On another busy call night, Emergency Medical Service
brought in a person from the streets. Frequently street people
are brought in the middle of the night, because they have
blacked out from alcohol abuse or are homeless. That night
they brought in a man on a stretcher with layers of dirt caked
on his skin. As they walked into the room where the male
patients wait for care, they happily announced to the emergency physicians, "We found this one in a garbage pail." I
examined the man the best that I could, but it wasn't until two
days later, after multiple baths, that one could see his skin. The
room by now was filled with homeless men, and the nurses
were spraying them all with lice disinfectant. All were crowded
into one room, without privacy other than for those few cubi-
cles separated by curtains.

Some homeless find shelter at Kings County. A psychiatry
resident told me that in the G Building, where the psychiatrists
work, the homeless are frequently allowed to stay in the waiting areas on benches. In the morning the guards wake these
"bench people," and out they go again onto the streets.

One man, well known to the medical community at Kings
County Hospital, comes in repeatedly, wearing a paper crown.
He's schizophrenic with a delusional thought disorder, but
harmless. He thinks he's the king of the entire waiting room
and of the emergency area. He sits on a bench, doesn't talk to

anyone, and walks around the waiting area as if to inspect everything. I see him less in the summer months and a lot around Christmas and during cold, rainy days.

The next day, as I left the hospital, I turned to gaze back at it. The Kings County Hospital complex, with its majestic buildings, detailed architecture, and colorful flowers, stands tall among the ghetto streets. This landscape hardly reflects the tumultuous activities within. I only hope that one day peace, opportunity, and good health will fill the lives of all.

A resident at Kings County Hospital must also rotate in a nearby community hospital, LICH (Long Island College Hospital). LICH has a mix of patients, for the most part they are upper middle class, and some poor. The hospital is situated in Brooklyn Heights and overlooks the Statue of Liberty, the New York Harbor, and Wall Street. At night, one can walk along the promenade of the community and get a breathtaking view of the Manhattan skyline glittering in the night.

During one of my clinics there, I remember a man with a syncopal disorder (blackout spells) who came into my examining room. He had only one layer of dirt over him. Apparently he had been a heavy drinker, and now he lived on the streets around LICH and in the park across from the hospital. I gave him a thorough examination. He wanted to be admitted in order to get a respite from the streets, but he wasn't ill enough for that, and I had to turn him away. The next morning, walking to work, I saw him getting up from the street. He was zipping up his pants and trying to make himself look presentable to the world as he prepared to survive another day in the streets. He wandered off into the park.

Toward the end of my first year at Kings County Hospital, I received a letter from my high school announcing my induction into the first Berner Hall of Fame. Nominations had been received from faculty, administration, other graduates, and the community at large. At the induction ceremony I saw many of the high school teachers who had given so willingly of their

time and their expertise in order that I might reach my goal of
becoming a physician.

I attained that goal and have become a physician and a neurologist, but I now feel myself confronted by new challenges in
the changing face of medicine today.

We must become involved. Medicine can no longer be practiced in an ivory tower, with the practitioner isolated from in-
volvement with the broader social and ethical issues existing
outside his or her own practice. These issues confront each of
us as citizens, and in many ways they control our practice of
medicine. We must, as physicians, help to establish more ex-
acting criteria as to what constitutes adequate health care. We
must be instrumental in passing legislation that will ensure that
these standards will be met. And we must become leaders in
guaranteeing adequate health care to all of our citizens—from
the very youngest to the elderly, the addicted, the victims of
AIDS, the handicapped, the homeless.

To the voice of the politician must be added the voice of the
healer.

# Chapter Seventeen

LOOKING back on my battles with cancer, I am glad that I am alive today to write this book, and that I continued to achieve my dream. Now I look forward to practicing neurology and toward stressing the importance of the human touch in our society.

I hope that this book will help people to believe in themselves and to forge ahead despite what appear to be insurmountable obstacles. One must not tremble in the face of forces that appear more powerful than oneself. Life is difficult, and there are hurdles to surmount. But they must be faced! Even after overcoming my disfiguring surgery, I still had to move back into society. Not everything had been sweet, and there had been real problems to contend with. Some people withdrew from me, others told me to conform, but still others had been there to encourage me to express myself.

You must live the life that was meant for you. Be true to yourself. Dare to be different. Share your ideas with others in active communication.

Driven with enthusiasm and a calling, I persevered through the rigorous training years of postgraduate medicine. I now look forward to inspiring others and to pursuing the clinical practice of neurology.

Neurology is an expansive field. Neurologists are diagnosticians who deal with many medically oriented problems—not only the ailments mentioned in this book but also problems such as headaches, backaches, slipped disks, sciatica, tremors and a wide range of other movement disorders, Parkinson's disease, dementia (including Alzheimer's disease), and painful or weak extremities.

As a physician, I focus especially on my patients' neurologic problems. Then I go one step further to see how that problem is affecting the way that patient is adjusting. Illness extends to all facets of a person's life, and those aspects, too, must be considered for a patient to receive the most effective treatment.

There is a great need for humanism in the world. This need encompasses all fields. Technology and the human element should work together for the benefit of all.

My wish is to see handicapped people helped by love, positive thinking, increased programs, and a caring public. Society must open doors to the handicapped and be concerned with their problems. The handicapped must play an active role in our society. People who are different should not be shunned.

The casual observer cannot see my facial deformity, but it is there: the widened left eye, the decreased facial folds on the left, and the separation between my crowned teeth and my prosthesis. My hearing is immensely improved, and a slight sense of smell has returned. My vision is nearly perfect, but my left eye, with more cornea exposed, still suffers from the harsh winds and cold. My head aches before storms. I still remove my prosthesis each night, and then I cannot speak. Also, during the day, I must remove it for cleaning after meals. I have skillfully concealed the leakage of fluid through my nose by carrying a tissue wherever I go. To the average person, it looks as if I have a constant cold. In reply to questions, I say that it is my allergies. I still need prosthetic adjustments and medical check-ups.

I address my new friends as the person I am; I no longer find myself making excuses for who I am. No longer do I tell them about my handicaps, although at times an occasional astute observer makes note of a facial asymmetry.

I don't become dismayed and wallow in self-pity. Instead, I forge ahead with the hope that I will help others as I have been helped. I want to encourage them by saying, "Believe in your dream; image it, and persevere. The victory will be yours."

# Chapter Eighteen

DURING my first year out of residency I was fortunate to be recruited into the New York City hospital system. As an Assistant Professor of Neurology with the New York Medical College, I spend most of my working day on staff, training other physicians at Metropolitan Hospital. I also teach at Lincoln Hospital and at the Westchester County Medical Center. In addition to these hospitals, I have staff privileges at St. Vincent's Hospital and Medical Center in Greenwich Village, the flagship hospital for Catholic hospitals. For the past two years I have also maintained a small part-time private practice on Manhattan's Upper East Side.

Contrary to much public opinion, the medical care afforded at our city hospitals is excellent, comparable in many ways to that of the big private hospitals in the city. At Metropolitan, we have a fine roster of physicians and an efficient networking system. All of our neurologists are board-certified, academic physicians; they regularly attend and/or give grand rounds, attend the annual meetings of The American Academy of Neurology, and keep abreast of the pertinent current literature in the field.

Unfortunately, however, Metropolitan and Lincoln hospitals lack some of the more sophisticated equipment, such as the MRI. (Magnetic Resonance Imaging is a new improved CAT scan.) Due to the high cost of such equipment, it remains the province of the more affluent hospitals. But the patients at Metropolitan and Lincoln hospitals can get access to the MRI at other hospitals.

One day shortly after I began work at Metropolitan Hospital, a female colleague asked me if I would like to become a member of the hospital's bioethics committee. "The other neurologist left and we need to replace her," she said.

I agreed instantly. Ever since my days as a humanitarian scholar at MCP and all through my medical training, I have cultivated a keen interest in bioethics. And my interest spans many cultures. For a short time I studied at Queens Square Hospital, London, and have toured hospitals throughout England, France, Thailand, and Singapore.

Bioethics spans issues such as life support, the right to die, organ transplants, health-care rationing, informed consent, treatment of AIDS patients, redefining death. The list of bioethical issues confronting medicine today is constantly expanding.

Indeed, new challenges will always confront us. Some will be met quickly and easily. Others will take longer. And still others may always remain with us. A new frontier is emerging—a frontier that will combine ethics, law, and medicine. Never before have these fields been so intertwined.

As a young physican today, I feel as if I am on the cutting edge of something new and exciting. My goal now is to be on the forefront of new issues as they arise, to champion causes, to become actively involved both in committees and in policy-making. And an important part of my future work will be to make the public as well as the medical profession aware of the new issues facing them.

The biomedical technology of today should be used as a powerful tool to protect our civil rights. This can be accomplished only through the education and participation of the medical community and of society as a whole. It is important to have an informed, enthusiastic public. Enthusiasm is the fuel that makes accomplishments possible.

The allocation of medical care and the economics of such care are becoming more complicated than ever. For example, it is no longer possible for a physician to open a private office without becoming involved with third-party payers and DRGs—Diagnostic Related Groups, an insurance billing and classification device whereby each diagnosis is automatically allocated a certain number of days for care in the hospital. If hospitals and physicians don't adhere to this set timetable, they are financially penalized. There is, therefore, a pressure both to admit and to discharge patients as rapidly as possible. Unfortunately, this may not always be in the best interests of the patient.

For example, a friend of mine who had become a patient in another hospital complex placed a call to me. He was frantic. "They're going to discharge me tomorrow. I'm not ready for it." His voice was almost a wail. "I feel so worn out, exhausted." His voice faded to a whimper. "How can they do this?"

I knew that this man had been discharged from and readmitted to the same hospital three times in less than a two-month period. Each time that he had been sent home, he was feeling almost as ill as when he had first been admitted. One time he was given a number of blood transfusions; another, he was admitted for congestive heart failure. On the third visit, he had been admitted for further testing and prostate surgery. Somewhere along the way, his blood sugar had skyrocketed and he had been introduced to a diabetic diet and given insulin instructions by a visiting nurse after discharge. Now he was about to be sent home again. In my opinion, he wasn't ready for discharge. But he hadn't felt able to present his case to the administrative body designated by the hospital to hear appeals from patients such as himself.

Why had all this pressure been placed on him?

Recently while on consult rounds, I was asked to evaluate a

seventeen-year-old woman who had developed a new onset of seizures. Two hours before my consult she had delivered her first baby.

As soon as I arrived at the labor and delivery area, I covered my street clothes with a yellow paper gown. These gowns are worn in order to prevent any spread of germs. Then I walked into her room.

The patient was sitting up in her bed, her newborn baby cradled in her arms. Her mother sat next to her.

I introduced myself and then asked, "How do you feel today?"

Her reply was enthusiastic. "I feel well, no more seizures. Do you know the results of my CAT scan?"

I steeled myself. "Yes, I do," I said. "Your scan shows an abnormality. At this point we don't know what it is. We must make more tests."

The patient's mother scooped the baby into her own hands and held it up to me. Her face beamed with pride. "This is my first grandchild—a grandson!" She exclaimed as though to impress upon me the fact that all must go well.

My heart ached. An hour earlier I had reviewed her scan together with my resident and the neuroradiologist. The radiologist had pointed to the contrast-enhancing abnormality on the scan. "It's consistent with toxo," he had muttered, visibly moved. He had pointed his finger at the film. "See the pattern of enhancement. I'm as certain as I can be without biopsy."

Toxoplasmosis (toxo) in a young person usually implies the presence of the AIDS virus. At our hospital we see all kinds of cases and, of necessity, must remain objective. But some cases pull at your heartstrings, no matter what. I knew that we would have to call the neurosurgeons in and do more studies in order to be certain of our preliminary diagnosis. But I also knew the skill of this radiologist. He was seldom wrong.

Now as I stood questioning the patient, she denied all risk factors.

"Have you ever had a blood transfusion?"

"No."

"Ever use IV drugs?"

"No."

I believed her. But that didn't make her prognosis any better. I knew that AIDS is increasing in the teenage population, mostly because of multiple sex partners and because of the sexual experimentation that goes on in that age group.

There is an ethical issue here. If the patient does have AIDS, then what responsibility, if any, does the health-care team have to inform the sexual partner? At this time, health officials are not permitted to give any information regarding the HIV status of an individual.

At present, in New York State, some physicians are trying to have legislation passed in order that AIDS can be treated as a communicable and sexually transmissible disease (Article 78 proceeding, entitled *The New York State Society of Surgeons, The New York State Society of Orthopedic Surgeons, The New York State Society of Obstetricians and Gynecologists and The Medical Society of the State of New York* v. *Axelrod*). This proceeding was dismissed by the Supreme Court in Albany County, but an appeal is pending. According to *News of New York*, a publication of The Medical Society of the State of New York, "With such a designation, public health measures to contain the spread of the disease can be undertaken." At present, there is no cure for AIDS. Prevention is our only hope.

On the other hand, those opposed to such a proceeding contend that fewer persons would consent to HIV testing if they knew that their confidentiality would be violated. They also contend that a person who knows his (or her) HIV status would probably confide in his partner(s) and that he would then most likely take some precautions. But if a person were not aware of his HIV status because he had refused testing, he might be less likely to take steps to alter his behavior.

The list of bioethical issues is endless. For the first time in my life I am in a position to address these issues seriously. This is the path that I believe my life will now take and I feel humbled by the great opportunities to serve which I am finding all around me. I find myself being guided into a study of the law in order that I may address these issues with the strongest voice possible. This does not mean that I will be giving up medicine. To the contrary. I intend to remain in my medical practice and to attend law school in the evening. In this way, I can also continue to participate in bioethics committees.

Halfway through the writing of this chapter I suddenly realized what a tremendous healing has taken place in my life. The realization caught me unawares, and it has been one of the most meaningful surprises of my life. Contemplating, writing about, all of my tremendous plans for the future, I suddenly thought, *Wow! There's not a word of personal illness in this chapter! This is an upbeat story, all about a young woman so filled with vitality, knowing she's going to make things happen.*

And then when I glanced back at the steps I had listed at the end of some of the chapters, I was awed to find that those best suiting me now were the "Steps to Shape a Dream" (Chapter Three). I realized that I hadn't been thinking of my handicap in relation to any of the plans that I had been making for the future. My handicap no longer stood out as something separate but in some way had been blended into myself so that I felt whole again.

Amazed, I examined myself in greater depth. When had this miraculous healing happened to me? I didn't know. I couldn't recall the last time I had thought of myself as handicapped. True, I still had the long dental visits to contend with, and some additional prosthetic work to be completed, but I didn't view these with the distaste and horror of the past. They had become a normal part of my living, and I had accepted them as such.

And I was surprised, too, to find that I held no resentment in my heart for anyone. I had so truly released any person whom I might have resented that I hadn't even been aware of that release until I questioned myself.

My romantic and social life has also been restored. Perhaps

not to the same degree that it might have been, but enough. This past week I had to turn down four invitations, three with eligible bachelors and one with a girlfriend. I was just too busy getting this book ready for the publisher. What more can a young woman ask?

And so, once more, I will follow my "Steps to Shape a Dream"; I hope that you will follow them too:

*Focus upon your goal*
*Plan your life*
*Develop your potential*
*Be willing to sacrifice and work*
*Exercise self-discipline*
*Be true to your convictions*
*Seek challenges*
*View problems from many different perspectives*
*Develop self-confidence; believe in yourself*
*Recognize the joy in each day*
*Inspire others to share your dream*
*Persevere*

God bless!

# Chapter Nineteen

TODAY I have at last regained acceptance as a "normal" person. Even more important, perhaps, is that I have been able to accept myself as normal.

I still have, and will always have, constant obstacles to overcome because of my handicap; a fine line separates the sophisticated, capable young woman from the severely impaired person. But it is with faith and positive imaging that I hang in and climb back up each time to the "normal" world.

Many of my patients, too, face or have faced seemingly insurmountable odds. My own experience with suffering, illness, and continuing rehabilitation has helped me appreciate and *practice* a humanistic approach to medicine. I am grateful that I can touch lives as a compassionate healer.

Eight years after my surgery at Yale, I was on night call as an attending neurologist at Metropolitan Hospital in Manhattan. The phone rang.

My resident's voice, urgent on the other end of the line,

alerted me instantly. "Doctor Engstrand! Come quickly! It's an
emergency!" he stammered. Quickly he sketched a brief history. ". . . unknown woman . . . beaten and raped several
times in Central Park . . . arrived by ambulance . . . b.p. 80
over palp . . . body temperature cold, 80° . . ." She had been
exposed to the elements without clothes, and was found half
submerged in the water of a nearby pond. The words poured
out of him in little staccato sentences. "She's in a coma. Her
pupils are fixed and dilated. She's on a respirator. They want a
neurologist to see her."

My mind snapped into action. "Treat her for herniation," I
said. "I'm on my way."

Minutes later I arrived at the S.I.C.U. (Surgical Intensive
Care Unit) and entered the room of an unknown female. This
then-unknown woman was to command national media attention. She was the Central Park Jogger.

By her side hung IV bottles, tubes dangled everywhere, and
a multitude of doctors crowded around her bed. "We're glad
you're here," they said.

I peered around the room at all the commotion. "What's
going on?"

The surgeon in charge of the S.I.C.U. turned from the patient
to look at me. "She's lost a lot of blood. We must find the
source of her bleeding."

An extensive evaluation revealed that a lot of her blood loss
came from severe scalp lacerations. From them blood oozed,
drenching her blond hair. Her left eye deviated to the left, and
black-and-blue tissue framed her eyes.

I grabbed my penlight and shone it into her eyes. Her pupils,
formerly fixed, were now sluggishly constricted, a sign that she
was starting to respond to emergency measures. I ordered the
appropriate neurological medications for her management.

A team of physicians including, among others, neurosurgery, neurology, psychiatry, and surgery was assigned to her
case. A CAT scan had revealed cerebral swelling and two blood
clots, one on each side of the brain. We opted not to drain the

blood clots but to monitor her intracranial pressure and to continue with conservative treatment. She was too unstable to undergo major surgery. Our hope was that the blood clots would get resorbed and that, as they did, the swelling would decrease and her condition would ultimately improve.

Some time later, when I was about to leave the patient's room, a resident interrupted my thoughts. "Dr. Engstrand, do you think that she will survive?" Enthusiasm usually sparked this resident's work, and even now, as I looked at him, his face held a look of anticipation.

It's good, I thought, that he's so eager to learn. I knew that he looked to me for guidance and that the way I answered him now might influence the way he practiced medicine not only now but also in the future. This medical team, I thought to myself, like any other team trying to overcome difficult odds, needs a boost in morale. "Yes, I do think she will survive," I said slowly, deliberating. "Where there is life, there is hope. Her pupils now respond. However," I cautioned, "it's too soon to tell for sure."

Just then one of my colleagues, though not on our patient's team, joined us at the nurses' station. His eyes focused on me. "I overheard your conversation and I disagree with you," he said, not unkindly. "The girl doesn't have a chance. Look at her!" He pointed to the little room enclosed by windows where she lay, and proceeded to analyze the case. The low blood pressure and crushed windpipe had starved her brain for oxygen over an extended period. His voice rose. "I want to instill depression into you. Face the facts now! It will make it easier for you later on. . . . If she survives, she could be a vegetable."

A *vegetable!* The word repeated itself over and over in my mind. This woman was only in her twenties, already an investment banker in a major Wall Street firm.

There are always two approaches to every problem in life: a positive one and a negative one. I believe that by adopting a positive attitude, one activates the wheels of good fortune. I knew that my colleague's opinion was both direct and honest,

calling the shots as he saw them even though he was not re-
sponsible for her treatment. My voice was cool as I defended,
nevertheless, the possibility of a favorable prognosis.

"Her pupils responded to treatment," I said doggedly. "Perhaps her exposure to the cold decreased her metabolic rate so
that her brain could survive with less oxygen. At any rate, it's
too soon to tell which direction her course will take. Why always look to the negative?"

"I don't believe in false hope," he said bluntly.

Nor do I. To me, false hope is a contradiction. Either you
have hope, or you don't. And hope based upon unshakeable
faith is the strongest force in the world. Such faith can move
mountains of despair and sickness.

Later that same day I revisited the Jogger's room. By this
time, the authorities had identified the woman, and her family
had been notified. As I approached her room I saw her mother
standing by her bed. I introduced myself as the consultant
neurologist.

"It's all so dreadful," she said, her voice a half-whisper. "The
first thing that I did when I met my daughter in this battered
condition was to make a joke of her bruised eyes. 'You won't
need eye shadow anymore,' I said to her." Her voice broke.
"How could I joke about that? I feel awful."

I looked away from her for a moment, remembering how my
mother had read joke books to me in the hospital, remembering
how, at a moment in my hospital room when all had seemed so
bleak, she had looked into my eyes and laughed—just
laughed—until both of us were laughing together when the
nurse came back into the room.

My mother had learned of laughter's healing power from
Norman Cousins's *Anatomy of an Illness*, and she had laughed
heartily on every possible occasion. And she had encouraged
me to laugh, even though my mouth and cheeks were immo-
bile and the laughter could take place only in my mind. Even
with my face bandaged, my eyes sewn shut, laughter was never

out of place. Mom had laughed, and the sound of her laughter had eased my pain and my despair.

Remembering, I knew what this woman needed to hear.

"Don't be ashamed to laugh," I said. "Laughter is important. It changes the mood of a situation and may even stimulate natural healing processes."

I studied the room critically. It seemed somber and drab. "Do everything you can to cheer things up," I said. "Bring in your daughter's favorite cassettes. Read aloud from joke books. Talk to her even though she cannot respond and, *very important*," I emphasized, remembering again, "be careful what you say in her presence. No one knows for certain what an unresponsive person understands." As I turned to go, I smiled warmly at her. "And do something for yourself too," I said. "Read Norman Vincent Peale, especially *Positive Imaging*, and Norman Cousins, *The Anatomy of an Illness*."

She studied me thoughtfully, near tears. "Thank you," she said.

One day, soon after the Jogger's admission, an old boyfriend brought in a photograph that had been taken of her two years before—a shapely girl, wearing a bikini and smiling as she held an oversized beach ball. Suddenly I no longer saw her as a disfigured person; right from the start, that picture helped me to image the patient positively—as the pretty, vivacious young woman that she had been and, I felt, would be again.

At long last the Jogger came out of her coma, drifting in and out of consciousness. Through it all her family encouraged her, told jokes, played her favorite music, and over time she began to respond to therapy. Each day I would ask her to squeeze my hand. Eventually she performed commands repetitively, gradually increasing her comprehension.

There were setbacks, but despite them, the staff of Metropolitan Hospital persevered, and we celebrated the little victories: the Jogger wrote her name, wore her sneakers, walked a few steps. We encouraged her to laugh and to see visitors.

Daily, she underwent memory testing. When she forgot things, she would become frustrated, but we encouraged her to keep trying. In order to build her confidence, we focused her attention upon things that she knew well. We knew that it was important to be aware of her needs in order that we might encourage her to fully develop her potential. We would start with her strong points, go back to the familiar, and then proceed from there.

During all of this time, no one dared to tell her what had happened to her. She herself did not address the issue. But suddenly one day she cupped her head between her hands in a futile gesture. "Something has happened to my head," she said. "There is something wrong with me."

"You're getting better," we reassured her.

Gradually she learned again to walk, to write, to speak. Even though she still lacked the insight to know where she was going, she knew she wanted to go somewhere. She was not yet capable of long-range goals, but she had a burning desire to live. She had always been a person with a purpose, and as soon as her strength started to return, she longed to do the things she had done before the attack.

Through all of this, the kinetics of active support from family and friends helped to keep her motivated. Strangers offered their support and love. Much of New York rallied around her, offering prayers and services. Letters poured in from across the nation. Her employer visited daily, serving as an umbilical cord to the outside world, helping her to maintain her identity. Cardinal O'Connor visited often.

And throughout the entire ordeal, her family never complained, never asked why this had happened to them. Instead, they united to help her, picked up the pieces, forged ahead with optimism. I encouraged them to take some time off for rest. If they became totally exhausted, she would sense it. She needed their strength.

Eventually the Jogger was stable enough to be transferred to a rehabilitation facility. Months later she returned to work.

*   *   *

So many people go through life hoping that nothing bad will befall them. But, the truth is that at some time in their lives, most people will face seemingly insurmountable odds: strokes, trauma, disease, bereavement, death. And it is to better cope with these times that it is vital not to fall into an apathetic acceptance of destiny. Character development and the nurturing of faith are almost a form of preventative medicine, an investment in a spiritual bank account. Make regular deposits into it of scripture, positive thinking, and meditation—in both good times and bad. That storehouse of faith will then be ready for you to draw upon when you need it the most.

Looking back on my battle with cancer, I am grateful that I am alive and well today, and I hope that my story will inspire others to forge ahead despite what appear to be insurmountable obstacles. I did it, and you can, too! Persevere. Recognize—and hold on to—the reality of your dreams.